Research Handbook for Health Care Professionals

Research Handbook for Health Care Professionals

Dr Mary Hickson
Therapy Research Facilitator in the Therapy Services Division
Imperial College Healthcare NHS Trust

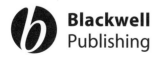
Blackwell
Publishing

Blackwell Publishing was acquired by John Wiley & Sons in February 2007. Blackwell's publishing programme has been merged with Wiley's global Scientific, Technical, and Medical business to form Wiley-Blackwell.

Registered office
John Wiley & Sons Ltd, The Atrium, Southern Gate, Chichester, West Sussex, PO19 8SQ, United Kingdom

Editorial office
9600 Garsington Road, Oxford, OX4 2DQ, United Kingdom

For details of our global editorial offices, for customer services and for information about how to apply for permission to reuse the copyright material in this book please see our website at www.wiley.com/wiley-blackwell.

Library of Congress Cataloging-in-Publication Data

Library of
Hickson, Mary, 1966–
Research handbook for health care professionals / Mary Hickson.
p. ; cm.
Includes bibliographical references and index.
ISBN-13: 978-1-4051-7737-5 (pbk. : alk. paper)
ISBN-10: 1-4051-7737-3 (pbk. : alk. paper) 1. Medicine–Research–Methodology. 2. Medical writing.
I. Title.
[DNLM: 1. Research Design. 2. Writing. 3. Evidence-Based Medicine. 4. Health Services
Research–methods. W 20.5 H631r 2008]
R850.H47 2008
610.72–dc22
2007047502
A catalogue record for this book is available from the British Library.

Set in 10 on 12.5 pt Palatino by SNP Best-set Typesetter Ltd., Hong Kong
Printed in Singapore by Fabulous Printers Pte Ltd

1 2008

Contents

Introduction

Why I wrote this book

I have been involved in research throughout my career as a dietitian; in fact my first job after qualifying was to run a research study. I then spent several years developing my clinical skills, before I came to the point within my work where I was faced with questions that I wanted to answer, and I was in a position to do so. I started with hesitant steps on the research pathway, my goal being to find information that would inform my practice and improve the care I gave to patients. My research career really began with a job running a randomised control trial, which enabled me to work towards a PhD. This gave me a grounding in the research process with hands on experience, as a PhD is designed to do. My job now is all about helping others to do research, and developing research capacity and capability within all therapy groups in the Imperial College Healthcare NHS Trust. This book has come from my experiences of teaching and supporting others who are new to research and those with some experience.

One of the best things about research is that I am constantly learning, developing skills and being faced with real challenges. Looking back on my career and research experiences I feel that there is a need for greater guidance for novice researchers. Of course, the people around me gave excellent support, guided me to the numerous detailed quality texts available for many of the individual stages in research (research methods, statistical analysis, writing skills), and directed me to suitable sources of information. Nevertheless, I would have really valued an overview of the whole process. Not everyone is in an environment that nurtures research and so I have aimed to write a book that can act as a guide, keeping researchers focused on the process and steering them towards further resources.

The purpose of this handbook and who it is for

This handbook aims to provide a starting point and a helping hand to guide you through the whole research process step by step. It introduces research in a practical and user-friendly way to student and qualified health professionals. It is primarily aimed at those people completely new to research, but experienced researchers will find many new tips and useful reminders. The handbook also provides a reference to the vast array of resources available for the researcher, and directs you to many other potential sources of more detailed information. So if you are leading, managing or co-ordinating research this handbook will provide you with a starting point for advising researchers.

Most text books distinguish clearly between the two philosophical approaches to research, concentrating on either quantitative or qualitative methodology. Although my roots are in quantitative research, I have learnt and used qualitative methods. Both approaches are valuable, answering completely different types of question. The important thing is to choose the appropriate research methodology for the issue you are exploring. This book incorporates guidance on both approaches to research and is therefore useful for science and social based health professions.

How to use this book

Experienced researchers or those managing research can dip in and out of this book; each chapter stands alone and can be used in isolation. Links to information in other chapters are made clearly.

If you are new to research you will need to start at the beginning and work your way through. I have divided the research process into three distinct phases: planning, doing and disseminating, and each chapter takes you through one part of these phases.

Throughout the book examples are included to help illustrate the processes or issues discussed. The aim of this book is to be a quick guide to the research process which you can use again and again over the years as you develop your research skills.

What this handbook cannot do

Research is a complex process that requires many different skills, and knowledge of specific regulations and procedures. This handbook cannot replace the valuable exchange of knowledge, skills and experience that accompanies one-to-one advice, and I would urge all novice researchers to find support from experienced people within their field or organisation. The handbook is a starting point to provide background information, to help you gain an understanding of the basic concepts involved and to facilitate a smoother journey into the wonderful world of research.

There are many other excellent texts currently available to help you through the individual stages of the research process, and many of these are listed in the resource section of each chapter. No single book can teach you everything and it is important to read widely and gain your knowledge from a variety of sources.

It is also important to remember that many procedures relating to research are locally agreed and as such this book can only offer a guide. Each organisation or NHS Trust will have specific policies and procedures, varying resources and a different focus on research. You will need to familiarise yourself with how your organisation operates.

Health research is dynamic and developing and so there is a constant need to update and review all parts of the research process; this handbook will be no exception. Please note that all the web-site addresses were checked in September 2007 and were accurate at that time. Also beware that information on the internet can be changed and updated at any time and so the author takes no responsibility for the quality of the information on the listed sites.

Acknowledgements

I would like to thank the following people who have provided advice, comments or simply lots of encouragement:

My colleagues at Imperial College Healthcare NHS Trust including Gary Frost, Jo Partington, Caroline Alexander, Davina Richardson, Rodney Gale and many of the staff in Therapy Services whom I help as part of my job. In particular I thank Davina Richardson for her help with the sections relating to qualitive research.

Judy Lawrence, Kevin Whelan, Julie Lanigan, Anne Holdoway and other members of the British Dietetic Association Research Committee.

Members of the Allied Health Professions Research Forum.

Members of the Dietitians Research Network, in particular Miranda Lomer.

Debbie Snell, Ailsa Brotherton, Elizabeth White, Kate Radford, Alison Culkin, Anna Horwood and Emma Kehoe for recommending specific resources.

The anonymous reviewers of the book proposal.

Finally, I would like to thank my husband, Chris, for his patience, support and his time spent proof reading, and without whom this book would have not been finished.

Part 1 Getting started and planning your research

The first phase of any research project is to plan exactly how you will carry it out. Good and thorough planning will pay huge dividends when you come to collect data and do analysis. It is important to understand that this phase will take many months, but it is worth doing properly to ensure your final results will be of value and merit publication.

Chapter 1 will help you think through the feasibility of carrying out research where you work, and Chapter 2 gives you a background to how research is governed within health care. The ten chapters following take you step by step through each stage of the planning process.

1   **Taking stock**

This first chapter should help you assess whether research is for you. Research requires certain skills and it is not for everyone. It is worth thinking through what skills you have, what support is available and how much backing your organisation can give.

1.1 What is research?

Research is the systematic investigation of a specific question in order to establish new facts and draw new conclusions. It involves the discovery of new knowledge and the interpretation and revision of current knowledge.

The process involves asking a question; collating and integrating current knowledge on the topic; designing a method to collect information to inform the research question; and finally developing new conclusions from the evidence.

1.2 Who does research?

Evidence-based practice is encouraged throughout medicine and related professions in order to ensure the treatments and processes we use are sound. Research provides the evidence. Involvement in research can be at various levels. Every health professional should be able to use research; in other words, find and critically appraise the work of others and decide whether it provides enough evidence to change practice. To achieve this some level of research training is given to all health professionals and many students are required to carry out small research or audit projects to practise these skills.

Getting more involved in research could mean helping carry out a research project; perhaps by providing clinical expertise to inform part of a larger project. This would mean that more experienced researchers will lead the project but it will provide an opportunity to start to learn the processes involved in research.

The next level would be to become part of a research team to develop a project, find funding and carry it out. More experienced clinical staff may find research at this level attractive since it offers a method to find answers to problems and improve patient care.

Finally, some health care professionals may wish to pursue a research career in parallel with, or instead of, their clinical career. To do this, a PhD is a minimum requirement, but this qualification could open doors to academic careers, leading research programmes, or teaching others.

The majority of research activity and support tends to be concentrated in larger NHS trusts and particularly in those departments with strong links to universities and teaching students. Nevertheless, research can be successfully carried out in any part of the health service if you have the will and drive to make it happen.

Universities are also centres of research and most successful health researchers will either work for, or have strong links with, a university. Health research is also carried out by commercial organisations and many charities are involved in funding and commissioning research.

1.3 Why should I do research?

All health care professionals are duty bound to provide care that is based on the best evidence available, which demonstrates that the particular therapy, intervention or technique actually works. Not all people are inspired to undertake the task of discovering new evidence, but all health professionals do need to understand how research is done and how to interpret the findings of others. Much of the first part of this handbook will help guide anyone through the process of finding, appraising and interpreting research. Other people will find the challenge of discovery appealing, and for those, the rest of the handbook will offer guidance on how to tackle the process.

1.4 What makes a successful researcher?

First and foremost it is important to realise that research is nearly always a team effort. Do not be seduced into thinking this means all members of the team share the workload equally; if the research is your idea and you are leading the project you will end up doing the bulk of the work. Nonetheless, having other more experienced people on the team means you can draw on their expertise and approach them for advice when you need it. This certainly means you will avoid many errors and it will also save you time. Since health care is often team oriented, there are many opportunities to link into ready formed teams to benefit from their experience and guidance.

Some of the characteristics a researcher needs are an ability to work methodically with attention to detail, good time planning and organisational skills, and an ability to communicate clearly. A good researcher also needs patience, determination, persistence and a thick skin to deal with rejection! Underpinning all of these traits good researchers must be curious, always questioning what they do, and they need to have a desire to pursue answers in the face of many difficulties. If you can identify with this description, research may be just the challenge for you.

On top of these personal characteristics, successful researchers need appropriate support from the organisation in which they work. This includes an environment where:

- research effort is valued
- time is allocated to undertake research activities including time to pursue clues and ponder
- researchers are permitted to develop a network of peer support through professional contacts both within and outside the organisation
- the researcher has appropriate autonomy or guidance depending on their experience
- team working is promoted to provide local supervision and mentorship

Published research suggests that overall it is having a supportive positive climate in which people can undertake research that has the most impact on research output and success (Bland & Schmitz 1986). You need to think realistically about the place where you work and consider how you will be supported and encouraged to pursue research projects. Try and locate researchers within your organisation and gain their help and support.

This chapter should help you consider whether you are in a position to pursue a research study or develop a research career in your current organisation. There are many transferable skills you can develop independently, but you also need to place yourself in an appropriate environment to really succeed. Research cannot be at the top of everyone's agenda and sadly this means some dedicated and enthusiastic people can be deterred from this career option; but if you feel research is for you, it is worth persisting and finding the support you need. Research makes for a creative, challenging and satisfying career.

1.5 Research, audit and service evaluation

While research is encouraged within the health service as a means to improve patient care and safety, it is not the only way to do so. The two main alternatives are audit and service evaluation. Although these two processes require some of the same skills as research they are distinct processes with different aims. Table 1.1 outlines the differences between the three processes in detail, but the single key discriminating factor is that of intent. The primary aim of research is to derive new knowledge; audit and service evaluation measure level of care. Research finds out what we should be doing; audit is to find out if we are doing it.

Table 1.1 Distinguishing between research, audit and service evaluation.

Research	Clinical audit	Service evaluation
Designed and conducted to generate new knowledge.	Designed and conducted to ensure the best care is provided.	Designed and conducted to define current care.
Designed to fill gaps in the knowledge base.	Designed to answer the question: "Does this service reach a predetermined standard?"	Designed to answer the question: "What standard does this service achieve?"
Quantitative research – hypothesis based Qualitative research – explores themes following established methodology.	Measures against a standard.	Measures current service without reference to a standard.
Quantitative research – may involve evaluating or comparing interventions, particularly new ones. Qualitative research – usually involves studying how interventions and relationships are experienced.	Involves an intervention in use ONLY (the choice of treatment is that of the clinician and patient according to guidance, professional standards and/or patient preference).	Involves an intervention in use ONLY (the choice of treatment is that of the clinician and patient according to guidance, professional standards and/or patient preference).
Usually involves collecting data that are additional to those for routine care, but may include data collected routinely. May involve treatments, samples or investigations additional to routine care.	Usually involves analysis of existing data, but may include administration of simple interview or questionnaire.	Usually involves analysis of existing data, but may include administration of simple interview or questionnaire.
Quantitative research – study design may involve allocating patients to intervention groups. Qualitative research uses a clearly defined sampling framework underpinned by conceptual or theoretical justifications.	No allocation to intervention groups: the health care professional and patient have chosen intervention before clinical audit.	No allocation to intervention groups: the health care professional and patient have chosen intervention before service evaluation.
May involve randomisation.	Does NOT involve randomisation.	Does NOT involve randomisation.
		Although any of these three may raise ethical issues, under current guidance:
Research requires Research Ethics Committee review.	Audit does not require Research Ethics Committee review.	Service evaluation does not require Research Ethics Committee review.

Adapted from National Patient Safety Agency leaflet *Defining research* 2007: Research, clinical audit and service evaluation.

This book is specifically aimed at those undertaking research; nevertheless many of the skills and processes are the same for doing audit or evaluation projects.

1.6 The stages of research

All research, both qualitative and quantitative, will fall into the three distinct phases; planning, doing and disseminating. Each phase includes several stages. A few of the stages may be optional; some research may not need funding, and statistics will not be needed for qualitative research. Figure 1.1 is a flow diagram of the process and illustrates how this book

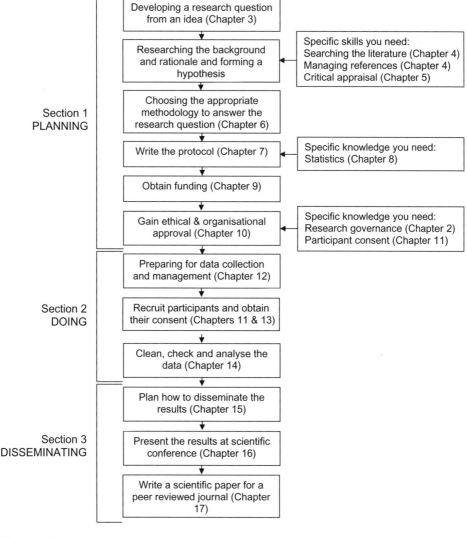

Figure 1.1 Stages of the research process.

links with each stage. This will enable you to use the book more effectively and gain an understanding of the bigger picture.

1.7 Resources

1.7.1 General information

To find out if you have a Research and Development Support Unit (RDSU) near you check: http://www.national-rdsu.org.uk/. RDSUs are funded by the Department of Health to support high quality and multi-disciplinary health and social care research.

RD Direct is the national advice service for researchers funded by the Department of Health and provides advice about the whole research process. Access at: http://www.rddirect.org.uk

For more experienced researchers this website may be of interest, which provides an online resource to support the leadership development of Principal Investigators: www.le.ac.uk/researchleader/index.html

Contact your professional organisation as many have a variety of mechanisms for promoting and supporting research activity, such as web downloads or library resources. For example, College of Occupational Therapy Briefing 75; Research Resources for Occupational Therapists (2007).

1.7.2 Information on the differences between audit, service development and research

Wade D. (2005) Ethics audit and all shades of grey. *British Medical Journal*, 330, 468. Available free at: www.bmj.com

Casserat D, et al. (2000) Determining when Quality Improvement Initiatives should be considered research. *Journal of the American Medical Association*, 283, 2275.

National Research Ethics Service, Defining Research 2007: National Patient Safety Agency, London. Available free at: http://www.nres.npsa.nhs.uk/docs/guidance/NRES_leaflet_Defining_Research.pdf

1.8 Reference

Bland, C. J., & Schmitz, C. C. (1986) Characteristics of the successful researcher and implications for faculty development. *J.Med.Educ.*, 61(1), 22–31.

2 Research governance

Before I begin to talk about the process of research I should first explain how research is managed and controlled in the UK. This should clarify, as you read through the following chapters, why some things have to be done in prescribed ways.

Research is vital for improving health care but does contain an element of risk, both in terms of return on investment and to the individual research participants. In order to ensure high scientific, ethical, safety and financial standards in research the Research Governance Framework for Health and Social Care has been developed. This describes how standards should be maintained, how decision making should be carried out, how research should be monitored and to clearly allocate responsibilities to all parties involved in the research process.

All research undertaken in the NHS or social care systems is governed by the research governance framework and the full details are available on the Department of Health website (www.dh.gov.uk – search for 'research governance'). Before undertaking any research you should be familiar with the research governance framework for the country in which you work. There is a separate framework for England, Scotland, Wales and Northern Ireland, but the frameworks all cover the same key topics. The governance framework is a guide for best practice and the details of how the framework is implemented may vary from organisation to organisation, so you must contact your R & D office for clarification.

The frameworks cover the following key areas:

- Ethics
- Science
- Information
- Health, safety and employment
- Finance and intellectual property
- Quality research culture
- The responsibilities of those involved in research
- Systems to deliver excellence in research
- Monitoring, inspection and failures

Many of these areas will be covered in more detail in other chapters, but a preliminary overview is given here.

2.1 Ethics

This section of the framework is wide ranging and includes: independent ethical review; informed consent; valuing patient diversity; patient confidentiality; data protection; use of tissue or organs; the use of animals; and involvement of patients in research. The guiding principle is that the dignity, rights, safety and wellbeing of participants must be the primary consideration in any research study.

The requirements for the ethical review of research and participant consent are covered in Chapters 10 and 11.

2.1.1 Patient involvement in research

Patient involvement is an area of increasing importance and all new funding streams in the National Institute of Health Research ask for specific information about this. Patients can be successfully involved in all stages of the research process at a number of levels. Patient involvement is about more than just consulting patients but also seeking to collaborate or even encouraging patients to lead the development of the research question and methodology. This can be a challenging area for researchers since traditionally, patients and the public have had little or no input into what health research is carried out in the UK and particularly in the NHS. Advice is available from INVOLVE (www.invo.org.uk), and they provide examples of how patients can be successfully included into planning research.

2.2 Science

This part of the framework aims to ensure that all new research builds on the learning of previous work and will add something new and useful to the body of knowledge once complete. Thus, adequate review of the relevant literature is vital. Reviewing the literature is covered in Chapter 4.

The framework also makes clear that peer review by experts in the relevant fields is essential for all research to maintain scientific quality. The level of peer review should reflect the size of the study and its inherent risks. For example, a large and expensive clinical trial is likely to need review by an external panel of experts, whereas small unfunded projects could be reviewed by one or two people within the organisation. The arrangements will vary locally but there should be a system for peer review available.

2.3 Information

This section of the framework covers the use and dissemination of information arising from the research. The general principle is that all results should be made freely available subject to appropriate scientific review, and also be in a format understandable by the general public. The framework recognises that there may be issues around intellectual property or possible commercial development of the results of research and allows flexibility in the timing of the publication of results.

2.4 Health, safety and employment

The framework emphasises the importance of health and safety regulations. You must make sure you are following all health and safety guidelines in force in your organisation. We are all responsible for our own and others' safety, and should act with this in mind. If you need to undertake any specific activity or procedure make sure you have been trained to do so in a safe manner, and understand the relevant health and safety regulations, such as regulations for working in a laboratory, taking blood, or operating equipment.

The *Research Governance Framework* says, 'A researcher not employed by any NHS organisation who interacts with individuals in a way that has direct bearing on the quality of their care should hold an NHS honorary contract.' (Section 3.10.3 of the *Framework* of England). It does not say every Trust must issue its own honorary contract, although in practice this is what tends to happen. This involves researchers going through an identical process several times in order to work in several different Trusts. This has been recognised as a waste of time and resources, so a researcher passport scheme has been piloted to avoid this duplication of information. Nevertheless, as yet there is no consistent approach, so you must check the local situation with your R & D or Human Resources Department. The NHS R & D forum may also provide helpful advice (www.rdforum.nhs.uk).

2.5 Finance and intellectual property

The framework underlines the need for compliance with the law and with the rules set out by HM Treasury for the use of public funds. It covers guidance on intellectual property rights, and it also covers the issue of indemnity against negligent and non-negligent harm to research participants, which is required to protect participants in trials. Research run within the NHS is covered by the standard complaints procedure, and the patient information sheet must include the indemnity procedure for the research. Sample wording is given in the National Ethics Research Service guidance (for website address see resources section).

If your research is being run in collaboration with an academic or commercial organisation there will be different indemnity arrangements. The National Research Ethics Service form asks for details of these, which you should be able to obtain from your local research services office or other management department.

2.6 Quality research culture

The framework recognises that although some parts of its guidance are clear and unequivocal, other parts require interpretation and judgement. In order to carry out high quality research that will meet all other requirements of the governance framework, strong research leadership and expert management is required. To engender an environment that will nurture excellence in research the following are listed as key principles:

■ Respect for participants' dignity, rights, safety and wellbeing
■ Valuing diversity within society
■ Personal and scientific integrity, honesty and accountability
■ Clear and supportive management and leadership
■ A culture of openness

2.7 Your responsibilities

The framework also outlines the responsibilities of each person involved in research and Box 2.1 lists the main people and organisations involved.

Box 2.1 Key roles and organisations involved in a health or social care research study.

Chief investigator
The person who takes overall responsibility for the design, conduct and reporting of a study if it is at one site; or if the study involves researchers at more than one site, the person who takes primary responsibility for the design, conduct and reporting of the study, whether or not that person is an investigator at any particular site.

Employing organisation
Organisation employing the chief investigator, investigators or other researchers. Employers remain liable for the work of their employees. The organisation employing the chief investigator normally holds the contract or grant agreement with the funder of the study. Organisations holding contracts with funders remain responsible for the management of the funds provided.

Funder
Organisation providing funding for a study (through contracts, grants or donations to an authorised member of the employing and/or care organisation). The main funder typically has a key role in scientific quality assurance. In any case, it remains responsible for securing value for money.

Investigator
Person responsible, individually or as leader of the researchers at a site, for the conduct of a study at that site. For clinical trials involving medicines, an investigator must be an authorised health professional.

Organisation providing care
Organisation responsible for providing health or social care to patients and/or service users and carers participating in a study. Health and social care organisations remain liable for the quality of care, and for their duty towards anyone who might be harmed.

Participant
Patient, service user, carer, relative of the deceased, professional carer, other employee, or member of the public, who consents to take part in a study. (In law, participants in clinical trials involving medicines are known as subjects.)

Principal investigator
The leader responsible for a team of individuals conducting a study at a site.

Researchers
Those conducting the study.

Research ethics committee
Committee established to provide participants, researchers, funders, sponsors, employers, care organisations and professionals with an independent opinion on the extent to which proposals for a study comply with recognised ethical standards. For clinical trials involving medicines, the ethics committee must be one recognised by the United Kingdom Ethics Committee Authority.

Responsible care professional
Doctor, nurse, social worker or other practitioner formally responsible for the care of participants while they are taking part in the study.

Sponsor
Individual, organisation or group taking on responsibility for securing the arrangements to initiate, manage and finance a study. (A group of individuals and/or organisations may take on sponsorship responsibilities and distribute them by agreement among the members of the group, provided that, collectively, they make arrangements to allocate all the responsibilities in this research governance framework that are relevant to the study.)

Reproduced with permission from the *Research Governance Framework for Health and Social Care* (England).

Each person or organisation listed has specific responsibilities described within the framework.

If you have developed your own project you will have the responsibilities of 'chief investigator' and 'researcher' (see Boxes 2.2 and 2.3). The terms 'chief investigator', and 'principal investigator' need a little explanation. The chief investigator is the person who is leading the research, but if the study is to be carried out over more than one site, each site needs a person 'in charge' who is termed the principal investigator. There is always a chief investigator but only multi-centre trials have principal investigators. However, some grant giving bodies refer to the lead investigator as the 'principal' rather than 'chief', which can get confusing.

The framework suggests that the chief investigator should always be a senior individual with experience; however, your own organisation will interpret this guidance locally. In my experience new researchers are perfectly able to undertake trials which involve a low risk to the participants, for example observational studies, interventions with no risk, or surveys, and may be the designated chief investigator. Where trials involve greater

---

Box 2.2 Your responsibilities as chief investigator can be summarised as:

■ Developing proposals that are scientifically sound and ethical.
■ Submitting the design for independent expert review.
■ Submitting the study (or proposal) for independent ethical review.
■ Conducting a study to the agreed protocol (or proposal), in accordance with legal requirements, guidance and accepted standards of good practice.
■ Preparing and providing information for participants.
■ Ensuring participants' welfare while in the study.
■ Arranging to make findings and data accessible following expert review.
■ Feeding back results of research to participants.

Reproduced with permission from the *Research Governance Framework for Health and Social Care* (England).

Box 2.3 Your responsibilities as researcher are:

■ Ensuring that any research you undertake follows the current version of the agreed protocol (or proposal).
■ Helping care professionals to ensure that participants receive appropriate care while involved in research.
■ Reporting any adverse drug reactions or other adverse events.
■ Protecting the integrity and confidentiality of clinical and other records and data generated by the research; and reporting any failures in these respects, or suspected misconduct, through the appropriate systems.

Reproduced with permission from the *Research Governance Framework for Health and Social Care* (England).

risk then it is more important that someone with experience takes overall responsibility for the trial. The framework has been developed to provide guidance and is subject to interpretation; the most important principle is the safety and wellbeing of participants and if there is minimal risk to the participants there is no problem with a new researcher leading the project.

The responsibilities of the other people and organisations involved are described in the framework document. It is useful for you to have an understanding of the responsibilities of others so you can appreciate why certain information and assurances are required from you and also what other systems are in place to support you as the researcher.

There are a few specific aspects from your own responsibilities and those of others that are worth highlighting:

2.7.1 Record keeping

If participants in the research are also patients, all relevant information should also be documented in the person's health record. In practice this does not mean all the information on the data collection form must be in the medical notes, but at the very least, the following should be included:

- A statement that the patient is on a study including the study title, a brief outline of what is involved and the date the patient was entered.
- Contact details for the investigator, including a 24-hour contact if appropriate.
- Ethics approval code.
- Any clinically relevant data collected that may influence patient care, such as blood pressure or weight. This should be updated at each visit if appropriate.
- Any changes to the patient's study status, such as that the patient completed the study, or has been withdrawn from the study.
- Any adverse events with the likelihood of the relationship to the study intervention (definitely related, possibly, unlikely, not related), and any action taken.

A label can be used to make it easier to include the right information consistently. Below is an example of a label used in medical notes at admission:

This patient has agreed to take part in the HIP PROTECTOR STUDY: (Ethics no. ••/••/••)

They are in the: (delete as applicable)
INTERVENTION group: They will be asked to wear hip protectors all the time during their stay.
CONTROL group: They will be treated as usual and will not wear hip protectors.
Date consented:
Physio signature:
For further information contact: Jane Smith: bleep 1234, ext 56789.

Researchers will also have their own set of records for all the patients on the trial, which should be kept secure, and will include all the data you need to collect. Treat these records as you would medical records; sign and date all your entries, deletions should be made by a single line and signed and dated; and everything must be documented. Records may be externally monitored and audited, and the outcome of such an inspection will impact on all the research done in the department.

2.7.2 Reporting and dissemination

This is regarded as particularly important within the framework. All projects should be reported at some level, even if the project has negative results. Information about your dissemination plan is also required for ethics approval and usually for grant application forms. The public must also be included in the dissemination plan, and this will require an alternative to a scientific paper. You may also need to communicate results to participants in your research, particularly if they request it. More information about dissemination and reporting your work can be found in Chapter 15.

2.7.3 Storing project information

All research data must be kept for 15 years, including data held on computers and paperwork. Data should be held securely, and it is advisable to develop a system for data storage within your department, so others can access the data if required in the future.

2.7.4 Conflicts of interest

It is helpful to keep a record of any funding or support you have received from any commercial company, at any time. You may be required to provide statements of possible conflicts of interest when publishing work or applying for funding. Examples of conflicts of interest that should be declared include:

■ Financial support to attend conferences
■ Support for a research trial in terms of money or equipment
■ Receiving an honorarium for speaking at conferences

2.8 Systems to deliver excellence in research

The framework goes on to describe the essentials of the systems involved in delivering high quality safe research. These systems will be the responsibility of the organisation. It will be useful for you to find out from your organisation the procedures that are in place and any policies that you are required to follow.

2.9 Monitoring, inspection and failures

The framework is clear that in the vast majority of cases, those involved in research will certainly adhere to the principles, requirements and standards of good practice set out within it. The incentives to do so are strong and include the law, the duty of care, and the need to maintain high professional and ethical standards. Nevertheless, mechanisms are required to monitor research activity and the framework goes on to describe how this should be done. Again, this section is largely aimed at organisations rather than individual researchers, and your organisation will have interpreted these guidelines locally. It is likely that at some stage in your career your project will be audited in order to monitor the research governance arrangements. Your R & D office will be able to give you details of local arrangements and it is worth bearing in mind that your work can be scrutinised at any time.

2.10 Resources

2.10.1 Websites

For copies of research governance documents listed below and further guidance access the Department of Health website (see the policy and guidance section > A–Z list > research governance):

- Department of Health. *Research Governance Framework for Health and Social Care*, second edition. 2005. London, Crown.
- Wales Office of Research and Development for Health and Social Care. *Research Governance Framework for Health and Social Care in Wales*. 2001. Cardiff, National Assembly for Wales.
- Department of Health, Social Services & Public Safety. *Research Governance Framework for Health and Social Care in Northern Ireland*. 2006. Belfast, Central Services Agency R & D Office.
- *Research Governance Framework for Scotland*. 2006. Edinburgh, NHS Scotland.

The Research and Development Forum is a network for R & D management in health and social care. They offer help particularly on issues of research governance – www.rdforum.nhs.uk

The National Research Ethics Service offers guidance on indemnity in the *Guidance on Information Sheets and Consent Forms* document, available on the applicants website under 'guidance' – www.nres.npsa.nhs.uk

2.10.2 Papers

Shaw, S., Boynton, P. M., & Greenhalgh, T. (2005) Research governance: Where did it come from, what does it mean? *J. R. Soc. Med.*, 98(11), 496–502.

Shaw, S., & Barrett, G. (2006) Research governance: Regulating risk and reducing harm? *J. R. Soc. Med.*, 99(1), 14–19.

Slowther, A., Boynton, P., & Shaw, S. (2006) Research governance: Ethical issues. *J. R. Soc. Med.*, 99(2), 65–72.

3 Formulating your research question

In this chapter I start my description of the research process by encouraging you to think deeply about the question you want to research. Initial research ideas are often very general, but good research questions need to be specific. That way you will be able to choose the right methods, identify the resources you need, pinpoint the criteria for success, and plan the work realistically to make sure the objectives can be met.

General ideas may flow from a range of desires:

- Improving therapy practice
- Understanding a problem in more depth
- Discovering the best way to treat a condition
- Determining how common a problem is
- Identifying people most at risk of a particular problem
- Predicting how a patient is likely to do
- Evaluating how a treatment works in routine practice

3.1 Be specific

In order to turn your idea into a question that can be researched, you need to be clear and specific on a number of issues, both clinical and practical.

3.1.1 Who are your target patients?

You will have a general idea about what patient group you are interested in but you may need to define more precisely who your patients are. This will enable you to develop the inclusion and exclusion criteria for your study. Some of the issues to consider are age group, the particular problem or behaviour, the length of time with the problem, other concurrent illnesses, social situation, and so on.

3.1.2 What is the problem?

You also need to be clear about the problem these patients have that you want to address. You may wish to try a new way of treating something, or simply gain a better understanding of the problem. Clarify exactly what you are trying to achieve by addressing this problem and describe your rationale for the proposed treatment or why this exploration is important.

3.1.3 How are you going to address it?

If you are testing a new treatment you need to be precise about what this will be and how it is different to what you usually do. If your research is about describing or exploring a problem, you need to think through how you will measure or observe what is happening.

3.1.4 Examples

The following three examples demonstrate how a general question can be clarified and in some cases this results in several questions which need to be researched separately. In each example the specific question describes the patient group and the problem precisely. At this stage the 'how' may be less clear to you.

Example 1

General: Does adding fish oil to nutritional supplements help COPD patients maintain their weight better?

Specific: Do COPD patients aged 60 years and over, who are underweight or have lost weight in the last 6 months, given 400 ml of complete nutritional supplement drink enriched with n3 fatty acids daily for 2 months, maintain their weight, compared to patients who take 400 ml of complete nutritional supplement drink without n3 fatty acids?

Example 2

General: Do patients with head injuries perform better in assessments of their function in their own homes?

Specific: Do patients with a head injury which affects their cognitive process skills perform better in activities of daily living when tested using Assessment of Motor and Process Skills at home compared to in hospital?

Example 3

General: Can attendance rates to physiotherapy outpatient clinics be improved?

Specific: What reasons do patients who are referred with lower back pain and initially agree to attend classes give for failing to attend the weekly outpatient class designed specifically for this patient group? By addressing these reasons can we improve the attendance to this class?

3.2 Be realistic

Once you are clear about what you want to investigate you must also evaluate whether it is realistic for you to explore it. Thus, you also need to consider the practical aspects of your research idea.

3.2.1 Where can this research be carried out?

You need to think through where you will have to do this work, and whether it is feasible to use these areas. Think about whether the research can be done within your place of work or whether you need to go elsewhere. Think about what facilities and equipment you need and whether you will be able to use them.

A study involving an intervention where patients may be seen several times over several months will have more implications in this area than a simple survey or questionnaire study. Whatever your study, think carefully about this factor as it will help you clarify what support or funding you need. Asking a few pertinent questions at this stage can save a lot of time later, and mean that you can alter the focus of your research to make it more achievable.

3.2.2 Do you have the time to do this?

If the answer is no, you will need funding. If this is the case you need to plan how and when you intend to obtain this funding, and more details are given in Chapter 9. Alternatively, what you propose may be entirely feasible within your job, or as a student you may be given specific times to do your project. Be very clear about how much time you have and when your milestone dates are.

For example, if you are a student and want to carry out research between October and March you will need to make sure preparatory stages such as obtaining ethics approval can be achieved before your start date. Alternatively, if you are working in clinical practice, your data collection may fit into your daily work schedules, but you might have to plan well ahead in order to achieve this.

3.2.3 Who else will need to be involved?

Research is nearly always done by a team of people, and so now you need to start thinking through who else should be involved. Who do you need in order to undertake and complete this project? What skills do you lack and where will you need others' advice and expertise? Have you got enough time or would it be better to work with others to 'spread the workload'?

Once you have thought thoroughly about your question and the practical aspects of research, you will have a sound basis on which to develop your detailed research protocol and project plan. This basic clarification is so important, but often people will rush ahead with a vague and undefined idea. Sooner or later you will have to stop and go through this process, otherwise your whole project plan will be woolly and incomplete. Such projects do not do well in obtaining funding and ethical committees will send you back to re-work your plan.

3.3 What next?

You should now have a clear idea of what you want to research and why, and who else needs to be involved. There are several other issues to think through, particularly if you need to apply for funding. You will need to justify why this research question is important, and explain how patients are likely to benefit from the work. At this stage it is essential to start talking to others to see if they agree with your ideas. It may be useful to approach your local Research and Development Office, a regional Research and Development Support Unit, your peers or experienced researchers in the field who may be able to help you. If you are doing research as part of a qualification clearly your supervisor or tutor will be able to help you, and the university may offer other general support.

Finally, you need to be sure your idea is novel. You need to review the literature to make sure the answer has not already been investigated. This literature review may cause you to adapt your question and will also help you decide the best methodology to use. I look at this subject in the next chapter.

3.4 Resources

RD Direct provides advice on question development at http://www.rdinfo.org.uk/flow-chart/Section1.htm, including a presentation entitled *Turning Ideas into Research Questions* by Jon Silcock, Leeds Teaching Hospitals NHS Trust.

The Research Assistant is an American website providing resources for behavioural science researchers. Much of the information is biased towards working in the USA but there is a useful section under 'Grant writing' about formulating a research question – http://www.theresearchassistant.com

4 Reviewing the literature

Now you have a clearly defined research question, you need to check that it is truly original, and to find out what related information there is that may inform the development of the study. The first stop should always be the National Research Register (www.nrr.nhs.uk), which contains details of ongoing and recently completed research projects funded by, or of interest to, the United Kingdom's National Health Service (NHS). It would be frustrating to do a lot of work on a project plan only to find someone else has already had the idea, and is doing the research.

This chapter discusses how to search the literature and provides an overview of the resources available.

4.1 How to search the literature

Performing literature searches is a skill well worth acquiring and honing. A brief overview is provided here to help you get started and further resources are listed at the end of the chapter. This section does not aim to teach you to use a particular search engine or database; but instead outlines the principles of good searching so you are better able to learn how to use the tools available to you.

4.1.1 Defining search terms

You already have your research question and from this question you can determine your key search terms. The more focused and precise the question, the more specific you will be able to make your search.

Your question can be formulated using the mnemonic PICO (Richardson et al. 1995), where:

P = Problem or patient: What is the problem or patient group you are interested in?

I = Intervention or exposure: What is being done to the patient or what possible exposure is of interest?

C = Comparison: What is the usual treatment or factor you wish to compare with?

O = Outcome: What is the desired outcome of the treatment?

For example:

Does bariatric surgical treatment improve weight loss in obese patients compared to lifestyle advice?
P: Obesity
I: Bariatric surgery
C: Lifestyle advice
O: Weight loss

All the terms you list under each heading will be your search terms and you may have more than one. In this example I could add 'gastric banding' and 'gastric bypass' to 'I' search terms. Table 4.1 shows further examples with different types of question, and that for some types of research not all categories are required. When deciding on your search terms within each

Table 4.1 Further examples of search term analysis using the PICO system.

Question	P	I	C	O
Does hydrotherapy treatment reduce the time taken to full function after an anterior cruciate ligament repair compared to land-based treatments?	Anterior cruciate ligament repair	Hydrotherapy	Exercise	Full physical function
How accurate is mammographic screening in the diagnosis of breast cancer in obese women?	Obese women	Mammographic screening		Diagnosis of breast cancer
What are the effects of drama therapy and related approaches as an adjunctive treatment for schizophrenia compared with standard care?	Schizophrenia	Drama therapy Psychodrama Role-playing Social drama group	Standard care	Mood Social interaction Psychotic sysptoms etc.
What is the prevalence of dysphagia in a hospital patient population?	Hospital patient population	Dysphagia		Prevalence

category think about the usual terminology, common alternatives, and alternative spellings for the most thorough searching.

4.1.2 Identify suitable sources of evidence

Virtually all papers published in journals are indexed on to electronic bibliographic databases, which can be searched in order to retrieve papers that match search criteria. There are two main types of bibliographic databases – secondary and primary.

4.1.2.1 Secondary databases

Secondary databases contain systematic reviews, summaries, guidelines and consensus statements. They all, in one way or another, summarise the available original research. The National Library for Health (NLH) (see Section 4.3.1 for further details) allows you access to several key secondary resources under the heading 'Evidenced based reviews', which are described in Table 4.2.

It is a good idea to start your search in these databases since this will provide you with an excellent overview of the current literature.

4.1.2.2 Primary databases

Primary databases contain the references to original research published in the journals covered by each database. Each database will be accompanied with a definition of what areas it covers and which journals are included. The most well know medical database is probably Medline, which is a general medical database with the emphasis on North American journals. Other databases include:

- Embase – Another general medical database, but with a greater number of European journals.
- AMED – Allied and Complementary Medicine – this covers many journals of professions allied to medicine and complementary medicine.
- Cinahl – This database includes nursing and therapy journals with a North American bias.
- British Nursing Index – This is a smaller database for nursing but with British and European bias.
- Psycinfo – Contains psychology journals and allied fields.

Each database has a slightly different content but there are vast areas of overlap between different databases. The most thorough search will include most of these databases but a more general overview of the literature can be obtained by searching two or three.

The databases are searched using search engines such as PubMed, Ovid, or Dialog Datastar. Each search engine enables searching of a specific selec-

Table 4.2 Details of the content and location of secondary databases.

Secondary databases	Contents
Cochrane Library www.mrw.interscience. wiley.com/cochrane	Provides high-quality, independent evidence to inform health care decision-making. It is often regarded as the gold standard for evidence. The Cochrane Library includes: Cochrane Database of Systematic Reviews (CDSR; Cochrane Reviews) Database of Abstracts of Reviews of Effects (DARE; Other Reviews) Cochrane Central Register of Controlled Trials (CENTRAL; Clinical Trials) Cochrane Methodology Register (CMR; Methods Studies) Health Technology Assessment Database (HTA; Technology Assessments) NHS Economic Evaluation Database (NHSEED; Economic Evaluations) A detailed description of each database is given on the Cochrane Library website (See 'More about the Cochrane Library' > 'Product Descriptions').
Bandolier www.ebandolier.com	Bandolier aims to find information about evidence of effectiveness (or lack of it), and put the results forward as simple bullet points of those things that worked and those that did not. Information comes from systematic reviews, meta-analyses, randomised trials, and from high quality observational studies.
Clinical Knowledge Summaries (CKS) http://cks.library.nhs.uk	This is an NHS funded resource that provides access to practical and reliable clinical knowledge about the common conditions managed in primary and first contact care. It helps health care professionals confidently make evidence-based decisions about the health care of their patients and provides them with the know-how to safely put these decisions into action.
Research Findings electronic Register (ReFeR) www.refer.nhs.uk	This is a database of the findings of research studies funded by the Department of Health and results are published here before publication. Thus, ReFeR fills the gap in access to research findings between project completion and publication.

tion of databases. The most well know is PubMed since it is freely available on the internet: www.ncbi.nlm.nih.gov/entrez. However, this only gives you access to Medline and for nursing, therapy and other allied professions it is usually important to search other databases.

For NHS staff the NLH provides access to Dialog Datastar which allows searching of all the databases listed above (see Section 4.3.1.3 for further details).

4.1.2.3 Which databases will give you the best answer?

Usually the first place to search would be the secondary databases for summaries of the primary research. If the information you are looking for is not there you need to choose the most appropriate primary database, which will depend on the topic you are searching. For a comprehensive search you should search several databases including both primary and secondary.

As you develop your literature searching skills you will become familiar with the content of each database and it will become easier and quicker to decide which databases to use. It is worth spending some time searching each database and exploring its content.

4.1.3 Devise a research strategy

You have your key search terms from your PICO analysis and have decided the most appropriate databases to search. There are two main ways to search databases: text word searching and using the thesaurus, and a comprehensive search will use both strategies. If you are doing a quick search to get an idea of what information is available, you may choose to use only one strategy.

4.1.3.1 Text word searching

Text word searching, as the name implies, searches the database directly for the word you type into the search box, and the search engine will retrieve documents containing that word or phrase.

Using text words, you are more likely to get unrelated articles and a larger but less specific retrieval. The search engine will only identify the exact word you type, so different spellings, misspellings and related words will not be picked up.

4.1.3.2 Thesaurus

In all the databases each entry is assigned a series of key terms that relate to the topics covered in the article. These have different names in different databases, for example; Medline calls them Medical Subject Headings (MeSH terms), Embase uses EMTREE and AMED calls them descriptors. These terms comprise the thesaurus for each database. They are hierarchical with major broad terms at the top of a 'tree', which are then sub-divided into increasingly specific terms forming the 'branches and twigs' of the thesaurus tree.

When using a thesaurus search you retrieve articles which have the specific term assigned to them. This avoids the text word problems of different spellings or terminology and hence the search is likely to be more specific. However, since each database has a different thesaurus you will need to search each individually, possibly with slightly different thesaurus terms.

In order to search using thesaurus terms you first need to choose the correct term by searching the thesaurus. Each search engine achieves this in slightly different ways but as an example PubMed has a MeSH database link on the left hand side of the home page. From here you type in your key word and possible MeSH headings are displayed, and you check the one that most closely matches your key word. However, to make things really easy PubMed automatically maps any text word typed in on the main search page to the thesaurus (MeSH terms). You can check which term has been chosen by looking in the 'Details' tab. For example, a text word search for 'elderly' is automatically mapped to the MeSH term 'aged' in PubMed (see Figure 4.1).

4.1.4 Search sources effectively

To make searching more sensitive and specific there are various tools you can employ. These include:

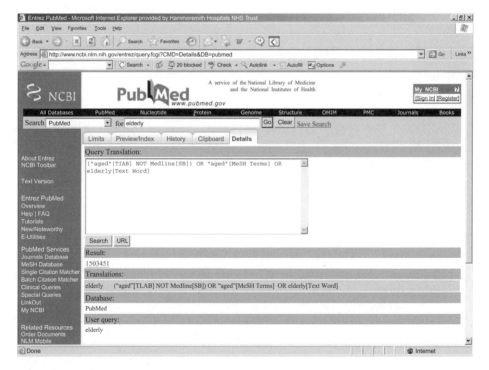

Figure 4.1 Screen print of the 'Details' tab showing how PubMed has automatically searched for the text word and the MeSH term (www.pubmed.gov – a service of the US National Library of Medicine and the National Institutes of Health).

4.1.4.1 Truncation

Truncation is a method that allows you to search for all words beginning with a particular stem. Most databases allow you to do this by using a symbol at the end of the stem to retrieve the range of different words with that stem. The symbol is $ (Dialog) or *(Pubmed/Cochrane), for example; Smok* will retrieve smoking, smoker, smokes, smoke in Pubmed, or depres$ will retrieve depression, depressing, depress in Dialog.

4.1.4.2 Boolean operators

These help you construct a strategy by combining, filtering or excluding groups of retrieved documents. The main operators to use are:

▦ OR – one or other of the terms must be in the document for it to be retrieved
▦ AND – both terms must be in the document for it to be retrieved
▦ NOT – will exclude documents containing this term

For example; if you want to search for articles about older people you might use the text words 'aged' and 'elderly'. If you enter into the search box: 'aged OR elderly' the documents retrieved will contain one of those two terms, but if you use AND both terms will have to be in each article for it to be retrieved. So in this situation OR is the correct Boolean operator to use.

There are several less commonly use terms (ADJ, NEAR, NEXT, SAME, WITH) available on Dialog Datastar and other search engines and I encourage you to explore them further.

4.1.4.3 Exploding thesaurus terms or using major descriptors

When using thesaurus terms you will get the option to 'explode'. If you choose this option it means that you will be searching for the specific term you have chosen, plus all the other terms underneath. This will result in a larger number of retrieved articles.

Alternatively, using the major descriptor option restricts your search to documents that have this term as one of the major descriptors and will not search for terms lower in the thesaurus tree. This will make your search more specific and smaller. An example of part of the Dialog Datastar thesaurus tree with the 'explode' and 'major descriptor' options is shown in Figure 4.2.

4.1.4.4 Limits

Different databases offer various options for limiting your search. These include restricting the retrieved documents to: English language only; a publication date; a certain type of study (e.g. reviews or randomised controlled trials) or human or animal work. Different databases provide

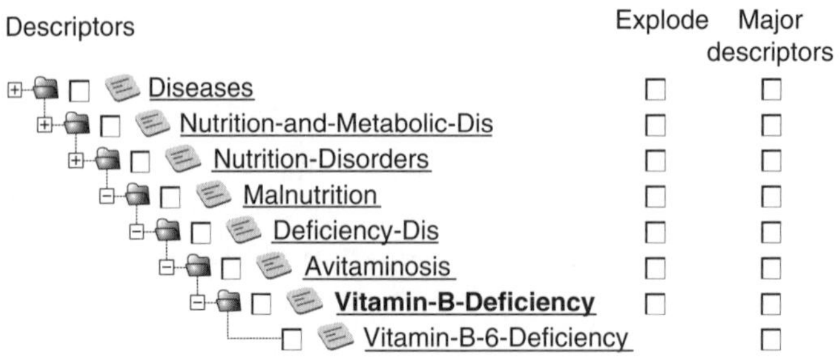

Figure 4.2 An example of part of the thesaurus tree from the Datastar Web system, to demonstrate the 'explode' and 'major descriptors' options. Ticking the 'explode' box for the term 'malnutrition' will search for 'deficiency disease', 'avitaminosis', 'vitamin B deficiency', or 'vitamin B6 deficiency' as well.

different options for restricting your searches, and you should fully familiarise yourself with them.

Most people do not have translation facilities so it is wise to limit searches to English language only. If you are undertaking an initial review of the literature you may wish to restrict your search to review articles to gain a rapid overview of the research area. If you are updating a literature review it is useful to put limits on the years to search.

4.1.5 Review your search strategy

Once you have done your search you will start reading through the retrieved documents to determine their suitability. You may find that you have far too many to look through, that many are irrelevant or you have only retrieved a few. At this stage you may wish to look again at your strategy and broaden or narrow your search using the tips given in Table 4.3.

Table 4.3 Dealing with irrelevant results or a limited retrieval.

Too many search results	Too few search results
■ Use major subject headings.	■ Use 'explode' for thesaurus terms
■ Don't explode terms.	■ Use text word searching as well
■ Look at the thesaurus tree and choose a more specific term.	■ Think of possible alternative words e.g. heart attack and myocardial infarct
■ Refine your search with logical AND and NOT terms.	■ Find a paper that is really relevant and look at the thesaurus terms used then search these.
■ Use the 'limits' options.	■ Repeat search on an alternative database.

4.1.6 Comprehensively searching your research question

To comprehensively search your research question you will need to be familiar with the techniques and tools outlined in the previous sections. You now need to plan a comprehensive strategy to find papers that will answer your question. To do this you will need to perform text word and thesaurus searches for each of your key terms defined in your PICO analysis. As you do searches they are automatically saved until you leave the search site. Then combine the searches for each section (P, I, C & O) using 'OR', which will result in large numbers retrieved for each section. Finally combine these searches using 'AND' to refine the final retrieval to only those articles which include all parts of the PICO analysis and reduce the retrieval to a small number of papers. Box 4.1 illustrates an example of a comprehensive search plan.

4.1.7 Store search results

Details of the retrieved documents can be saved and printed as well as uploaded into reference managing software (see Section 4.2). For specific

---

Box 4.1 Comprehensive search strategy for a specified research question.

Does surgical treatment improve weight loss in obese patients compared to lifestyle advice?

P: Obesity, overweight
I: Gastric bypass, gastric banding, bariatric surgery
C: Lifestyle advice
O: Weight loss

Search plan:

  1: Text word search: Obesity OR overweight
  2: Thesaurus search: Obesity OR overweight
  3: Text word search: Gastric bypass OR gastric banding OR bariatric surgery
  4: Thesaurus search: Bariatric surgery using 'explode'
  5: Text word search: Lifestyle advice or health behaviour
  6: Thesaurus search: Health behaviour
  7: Text word search: Weight loss
  8: Thesaurus search: Weight loss
  9: Combine searches using OR: search 1 OR 2
 10: Combine search 3 OR 4
 11: Combine search 5 OR 6
 12: Combine search 7 OR 8
 13: Combine searches using AND: 9 AND 10 AND 11 AND 12

On PubMed this retrieves 35 articles (unlimited by language or other limit, June 2007).

instructions on how to do this you will need to look for guidance in the help sections of the relevant search engine and in the software manual. Many search engines also offer the option to save your search history so you can run it again in the future.

4.1.8 Compiling a literature review

When you first start to look at the literature about a particular topic it is useful to start compiling a working document of all the reading you do. By a working document I mean a document that is for you not anyone else; it is a document you can add to gradually and develop as your understanding of the area increases. You can use your own shorthand and notes, you can write in whatever style works for you; the purpose of the document is to help you keep track of your reading and to summarise what the literature is telling you. When you come to writing a more formal document, like the research protocol, you can select the appropriate information from the working document, along with relevant references, quickly and easily.

The first step is to define your general topic area that relates to your research question. So for example; What is the prevalence of dysphagia in a hospital patient population? The general topic would be dysphagia and under this could come a variety of sub-topics relating to prevalence, identification and diagnosis, consequences, aetiology, and treatment. Clearly for this research question you will be most interested in prevalence and diagnosis, but the other areas will inform your work and give you a broader understanding of the current knowledge in the area. Each of these sub-topics will become a heading in your document. Under each heading you can start to summarise the information available; providing references and a critique of the papers' quality.

If you work better using visual representations Cresswell (2003) suggests the use of a literature map to start the process of a literature review. This involves drawing a diagram to show how the main topic and sub-topics link together and other areas that also connect with these topics. Such a visual aid can help you organise your thoughts and provide a structure for your working document.

4.2 Reference management

Keeping your references filed in a manner that makes them readily accessible is not easy. While doing literature reviews you can accumulate large numbers of paper and electronic copies of research articles and it is difficult to keep track of what you have read, what is useful and what is not.

I have no easy solution to this problem but I would strongly advise that you think through what will work best for you at an early stage. There are various software programs available to help you manage your references, for example: Reference Manager, ProCite and Endnote.

Most of this type of software can:

- Store your references in a database. You can have several databases, each for different topics.
- Download references from internet reference libraries.
- Enter references manually.
- Enter references by importing text files.
- Search internet based libraries, e.g. PubMed.
- Mark entered references to say whether you have a hard copy.
- Link the reference in the database to electronic copies of the whole paper.
- Retrieve references by searching any information you can remember about them like author, date, journal, key word or title word.
- Add references to text as you write papers or reports. The software will then create and format the bibliography and in-text citations according to any journal style.
- Create or modify journal styles if you need to.

This software will make sure your references are accurate and in the correct order and format. It is far more reliable than trying to do them manually.

In short, it is an invaluable tool to save you time and effort when writing papers, reports or grant applications – in fact anything where you need to add references to the text. It may take a little time to get used to it, but in the long term it will save you lots of time.

4.3 Making the most of the library

Most hospitals or primary care trusts have access to library facilities, and large teaching hospitals and universities usually have considerable resources. Find out what you have available locally and how to access it. Librarians are a valuable and often underused resource; they will be able to help you sort through which resources will be of most use to you and teach you how to use them.

4.3.1 National Library for Health

All NHS staff now have access to the National Library for Health or NLH (www.library.nhs.uk). Through this you are able to search a variety of databases, access some full text journals, access the Cochrane library and many other health information resources, download free medical images, keep up to date with recent evidence and guidelines, get summaries of the top health related news stories, search medical dictionaries and personalise your account to provide relevant updates, journal table of contents and links to websites of interest. Many of these resources are available to all, so even if you do not work within the NHS it is worth investigating this site.

4.3.1.1 Registration

To access some of the resources on the NLH you need to obtain an Athens password. Further information is available from your local library or online on the NLH website; click on 'register for Athens'. You need to be working or a student within the NHS, have a current email address and know the NHS region and area for the NHS organisation you are in.

4.3.1.2 Full text journals

The NLH has a collection of full text journals currently managed by TDNet. It covers both Clinical Science and Health Management. If you have an Athens password you can access these journals. You can search the full text collection using the 'My Journals' link, or indirectly via the bibliographic databases.

If you do not have access to NLH journals your organisation may sub-scribe to a different selection and if you are a student, your university will provide access to many journals.

4.3.1.3 Bibliographic databases

NLH provides access to a range of bibliographic databases including; Medline, Cinahl, Psycinfo, EMBASE, AMED (Allied and Complimentary Medicine), British Nursing Index, DH-data, and Kings fund. They can be accessed under the 'Resources' section and they are searched using Dialog Datastar.

Access to bibliographic databases is essential for good quality research. However, no single database covers all journals; and therapy and allied medical professionals in particular will find many journals covering their area are not on Medline. Nevertheless, Medline can be freely accessed by all using PubMed. See Section 4.1.2.2 for more information.

4.3.1.4 Clinical knowledge summaries

This is a source of clinical knowledge for the NHS about the common con-ditions managed in primary and first contact care. Its main function is to help health care professionals confidently make evidence-based decisions about the health care of their patients and provides the know-how to safely put these decisions into action. However, it also provides a very useful source of information for researchers performing a review of their topic.

4.3.1.5 Evidence updates

These include a health management specialist library, access to National Institute of Health and Clinical Excellence (NICE) guidelines and the Centre for Reviews and Dissemination.

4.3.2 *Keeping up to date with the literature*

There are various resources to do this via email and the internet. Several providers allow you to register a list of journals you are interested in, and you are then emailed the table of contents when they are published. With your NHS Athens user name you can do this on the NLH website, using the 'My Journals' link. Another provider is Zetoc (http://zetoc.mimas.ac.uk/), which may be available to you if you are in higher education. You can also register for tables of contents on specific journal sites, which can be more up to date than other secondary service providers. Ask at your library for more information or explore the options available on the NLH site.

4.4 Resources

Undertaking a comprehensive literature review is a highly skilled task. Anyone can do a quick and dirty scan through the literature, but to be confident you have retrieved all the relevant publications on a particular topic is a skill that requires practice and guidance. It is not an easy skill to develop and you need to be disciplined and think logically. It is highly advisable to obtain further hands-on training from your institution or from an experienced researcher or librarian. Many libraries will offer training and courses are often part of university degrees. Research and Development Support Units (www.national-rdsu.org.uk) or local R & D offices may also organise training. Dialog Datastar, PubMed and other search engines such as Ovid have useful tutorials and demonstrations.

4.4.1 Websites

The Internet also has numerous resources which are best located by using the search term 'searching medical literature' in any search engine. One example is Researching Medical Literature on the Internet – 2005 Update, by Gloria Miccioli (http://www.llrx.com/features/medical2005.htm). This discusses the various sources of information available and how to get the most out of them, but has a slight bias towards USA sites.

National Research Register – www.nrr.nhs.uk

Pubmed – www.ncbi.nlm.nih.gov/sites/entrez

National Library for Health – www.library.nhs.uk

4.4.2 Distance learning resources

Evidenced Based Health Care – A CASP CD-ROM and Workbook (http://www.phru.nhs.uk/Pages/PHD/CDROM.htm)

Certificate in Evidence Based Practice, Leeds Metropolitan University and the Scheidegger Institute. (http://www.scheidegger-institute.com/index.html)

4.4.3 Papers

Greenhalgh T. (1997) How to read a paper. The Medline database. *BMJ*, 315, 180–183.

Woods D., & Trewheellar K. (1998) Medline and Embase complement each other in literature searches. *BMJ*, 316, 1166.

4.4.4 Books

Hart, C. (1998) *Doing a Literature Review – Releasing the Social Science Research Imagination.* Sage, London – a thorough examination of how to undertake and produce a literature review. A book worth dipping into with lots of useful practical tips.

Rumsey, S. (2004) *How to Find Information – A Guide for Researchers.* Open University Press, Maidenhead – this is a comprehensive text to help you find the information you need.

4.5 References

Cresswell, J. W. (2003) Review of the literature. In *Research Design: Qualitative, Quantitative and Mixed Method Approaches*, 2nd edn. Sage, London, pp. 27–48.

Richardson, W. S., Wilson, M. C., Nishikawa, J., & Hayward, R. S. (1995) The well-built clinical question: a key to evidence-based decisions. *ACP J Club.*, 123(3), A12–A13.

5 Critically appraising papers

Critical appraisal is a technique for increasing the effectiveness of your reading. It enables you to quickly exclude papers that are of poor quality that will not inform practice or your research. For those papers that do come up to scratch, it enables you to systematically evaluate their strengths and weaknesses, and to distil their key findings.

5.1 How can it help?

Critical appraisal offers a way through the huge volume of material now being published. There are over 6000 journals on the ISI science journal citation report database (http://wok.mimas.ac.uk) and most of these publish hundreds of articles each year. Only a small proportion of these will be relevant to your particular field of interest, but nevertheless, there will still be numerous journals you could be looking in either monthly or weekly to keep up to date in your field. This will result in many papers that interest you but only a small number that will really change your practice. Critical appraisal helps you decide how applicable the research is to 'real life' situations and whether it will help improve your clinical practice.

Equally, when searching the literature for the background to a study you will find a mixture of good and bad studies; the bad studies are not helpful in developing your study protocol. It is important to evaluate the evidence already available when refining your research question and designing your study; additionally, funding bodies and ethics committee will certainly ask you for an evaluation of the published literature in your area. Critical appraisal will help you sort the wheat from the chaff.

5.2 How do I critically appraise research papers?

There is no one absolute method of critical appraisal; different people structure critical appraisal in different ways. The method presented here is one approach that many people have found helpful and easy to follow and is based on the Critical Appraisal Skills Programme (CASP© Milton Keynes Primary Care Trust 2002) and the Users' Guides to the Medical Literature published in the *Journal of the American Medical Association*. However, there are plenty of other resources available to guide you and some of these are listed at the end of the chapter.

There are three basic areas to consider for all papers:

■ Message: what are the main results and conclusions of the article?
■ Validity: can the results and conclusions be justified based on the description of the methodology and findings?
■ Utility: is the research relevant to the study I am planning? Will the results be applicable to my patients?

The specific questions you need to ask yourself about each paper will depend on the design and methodology of study you are appraising. Examples of the sort of questions you need to ask about a randomised control trial, a systematic review and a qualitative study, within each of the three major areas are listed in Table 5.1.

Table 5.1 illustrates that the main area for consideration when assessing the quality of the paper is the methodology. If this is sound the results are also likely to be robust and you can then draw your own conclusions before reading the discussion, to see if you agree with the paper's authors. The questions to ask about the validity of the paper vary the most between study designs but you should always start by looking for a clear and explicit research question or study aim. Further detail on questions to ask about other study designs (cohort, case control, etc.) can be found by using the resource section at the end of this chapter. The questions to consider about the utility and the message of the paper are fairly similar whatever the study design. More detail on how to identify different study designs is given in Chapter 6.

When you are reading research papers start by looking for the research question (hypothesis or study aim), which is usually at the end of the introductory section. Next work your way through the methods section by looking for the answers to the questions appropriate for the design. At any point, if the answers to these questions are poor, you need to consider whether it is worth continuing – Is this paper really going to tell you anything useful at all? Is it better to leave this paper and read another instead?

You are trying to use critical appraisal as a method to filter through the mass of literature available, so do just that. Be critical and be sceptical. If the information is not there, do not assume the research has been carried out in the best way. If all the results are not reported – perhaps it is because they do not support the hypothesis. Look for inconsistencies. Do not assume that just because it is published in a peer reviewed journal it must be useful. If you think the paper is not useful, leave it and move on.

Having emphasised the need for a healthy dose of scepticism, it is important not to take this strategy to extremes. Almost any human study can be

Table 5.1 Examples of the type of questions you need to ask about three different study designs.

	Randomised control trial	Systematic review	Qualitative study
Validity Are the findings valid?	■ Did the trial address a clearly focused issue? ■ How was the sample selected? Is it big enough (power calculation), and is it representative? ■ Was the assignment of patients to treatments randomised? ■ Were all the patients who entered the trial properly accounted for at its conclusion? ■ Was the analysis done on an intention to treat basis? ■ Are there any differences between the two groups that could explain the differences between them? (factors like age, sex, social class, activity, smoking etc) and were the groups similar at the start of the study? ■ Were the patients, workers, study personnel 'blind to the treatment'? ■ Except for the experimental intervention, were the groups treated equally? ■ How large was the treatment effect? (consider what outcomes were recorded, and how the differences between the groups were expressed) ■ How precise was the estimate of the treatment effects? (hint: look for confidence intervals).	■ Does the review attempt to answer a clear and focused question? ■ Have the authors done a thorough and comprehensive literature review, including numerous databases, other literature sources, and foreign literature? ■ Are explicit inclusion and exclusion criteria defined for which studies are included in the review? ■ Are the reasons for the excluded studies clear? ■ How was the quality of the included studies assessed? ■ If a meta-analysis has been done, was it appropriate and reasonable to combine the results of the included studies? ■ How are results presented? ■ What are the key results? ■ How precise are the results (look for those confidence intervals)?	■ Was there are clear statement of the aims of the research? ■ Was the design of the research appropriate to achieve the aims of the research? ■ Has the researcher explained and justified the design they have chosen? ■ How were the participants chosen and recruited? ■ Are these participants the most likely to inform the aims of the study? ■ Was the method of data collection explicit and appropriate to the research issue? ■ Has the relationship between the participants and the research been considered? ■ Has the researcher explored sources of bias? ■ How was the data analysis done and is this appropriate to the aims of the study? ■ Are sufficient data included to support the findings of the study? ■ Have exceptions and contradictory data been presented or discussed? ■ What are the key findings? ■ Are the findings adequately discussed and justified? ■ How credible are the findings?

Table 5.1 Continued

	Randomised control trial	Systematic review	Qualitative study
Utility How useful are these results for me?	▪ Can the results be applied to the local population? i.e. how different are the patients in the study population from those sitting in your clinic? ▪ Were all the clinically important outcomes considered? If any were neglected, does this affect the interpretation? ▪ Are the benefits worth the harms and costs? This is a bonus, as much research will not include cost benefit analyses.	▪ Can the results be applied to the local population? ▪ Were all the clinically important outcomes considered? If any were neglected, does this affect the interpretation? ▪ Are the benefits worth the harms and costs? You may need to make this judgement yourself since this type of analysis is not always included. ▪ Should I change my practice?	▪ How do the findings fit in with current knowledge and what do they add? ▪ Has the generalisability of the results been considered? ▪ Are new areas of study raised? ▪ Can this information change or inform my practice?
Message What is the message of the paper?	▪ What is the message to take back to clinical practice? ▪ What is the bottom line? ▪ How does this work support the research I am planning?	▪ What is the message to take back to clinical practice? ▪ What is the bottom line? ▪ How does this work support the research I am planning?	▪ What is the message to take back to clinical practice? ▪ What is the bottom line? ▪ How does this work support the research I am planning?

criticised in one way or another, so do try to take a balanced view and think about whether the research could have realistically been done in a better way. Think carefully about whether the flaws you identify are likely to significantly affect the final results before you reach a conclusion on the paper. Ideally, your approach to critical appraisal is one which takes a measured, balanced view. Walk a line between the extremes of assuming that every research paper is written by a pathological liar and must be torn apart, and the opinion that because papers are published they must be good and are beyond reproach.

5.3 Other things to think about

There are other aspects of study design and research governance that you may also consider as you review papers. For example, how would you regard the report of a project funded by a company who marketed some of the drugs or equipment involved? There is evidence of publication bias in pharmaceutical and nutrition research so this is worth considering (Bekelman, Li & Gross 2003; Lesser et al. 2007).

What about ethics? Would you use the results of a study where you felt there were ethical problems and no explicit evidence of Ethics Committee approval? Although many biomedical journals now require clear evidence of ethical approval before publication, evidence suggests ethical issues can still arise (Bauchner & Sharfstein 2001) and there is continuing debate in the medical literature about ethics in research.

5.4 Appraising the statistics

Critical appraisal of the statistics used in the research is important but many people find this daunting and have little confidence in their skills in this area. You do not have to be a mathematician to appraise the statistics but you will need an understanding of the fundamental principles of probability and risk assessment. Much of the fear induced by the statistics is due to unfamiliar terminology; tackling a host of incomprehensible jargon is overwhelming and difficult. Nevertheless, you have to start somewhere and take that first step to learning the terms involved. Chapter 8 has been written to get you started with statistics.

When reading and appraising papers start by looking at the description of the statistics used and try to understand why certain tests have been chosen (more on this in Chapter 8). Next focus on the main results (look for the primary outcome measure the researchers have used – see Section 7.2.6.5) and work through what the figures are telling you. See if your interpretation of the figures matches that of the authors. Next, look at the other data presented and see if they help explain or clarify the main results.

Finally, beware of 'statistically significant' results that are not 'clinically significant'. Statistical significance means that we can be confident the result is true, but clinical significance means the result will make a difference to the treated patient. For instance, a new physiotherapy exercise intervention compared to the usual practice may show a 'very significant' ($p < 0.001$) improvement in the 'timed up and go' test, but that difference may be only 3 seconds, which is unlikely to make much difference to the patients' quality of life. You will need to use your clinical expertise within your area to make this judgement.

5.5 Journal clubs

An excellent way to practise and develop your critical appraisal skills is to regularly attend a 'journal club'. Critical appraisal skills are not easy and take time to develop as you learn about different study designs and statistics, and refine your analytical skills. The more you practise the better you will get and the quicker you will be able to appraise a paper. The strength of a club is that you will learn together; educating each other and sharing the burden of looking up terms or unfamiliar techniques.

The general idea is that a group of people get together (such as your department or your multi-disciplinary team), choose a paper to appraise and then critique it together. A well run journal club that encourages participation from all is a stimulating and educational experience. However, journal clubs do have the potential to be very dull, a platform for some people to extol their expertise, and can be intimidating to quieter or more junior team members. With care this problem can be avoided, and I describe here a successful approach I have used with a number of therapy professions that has received positive feedback (see Boxes 5.1 and 5.2); this is not the only way and others have described a variety of approaches (Gibbons 2002; Gonzalez 2003; Higgins & O'Gorman 2006).

A schedule for the club is agreed and each person in the team is assigned a date to choose a paper they think would be either interesting or may lead to changes in practice. The chosen paper is circulated to the whole team prior to the club (at least one week before) and everyone is expected to read it. The critical appraisal skills programme tools (CASP tools – see Resource section) are used to help with the appraisal process, and each person comes to the journal club with a couple of questions in mind to ask others about the paper. The questions could be those listed in the CASP tool or it could be a specific issue about the paper.

The organiser for that week chooses one of their questions then picks one of the other participants to answer it. This person attempts to answer the question and engages others in the discussion. This person now asks someone else a question, and so the discussion continues encouraging all to participate.

Box 5.1 What do you think about this style of journal club?

■ It helps increase learning as you can ask questions to each other in a non-threatening environment.
■ Using CASP tools is an easier guide to critically appraise the paper.
■ It has changed from being a passive exercise to an interactive session where we not only keep up to date with current literature but also learn valuable appraisal skills and by having all read it we learn a lot from each other too.
■ I am getting more out of attending and see it as a valuable process, even if the paper is not in my topic area
■ I like it. I really do feel that I am learning from it. Hearing others' opinions often confirming your own, gives you confidence.
■ I feel like we are learning together as a group
■ I am motivated to read the paper because I know it will result in valid debate and discussion
■ Much more constructive way of spending my time. I enjoy it now!!

Box 5.2 What have you learnt?

■ I feel much more competent in analysing papers on a daily basis for my own work.
■ A lot more about stats, but still loads to go.
■ That reading a paper is not all that scary or difficult. That people may have very different views based on the same paper.
■ How to skim read a paper – it's not always necessary to plough through all the intro and discussion if you've read the method and results
■ Not assuming all studies are good just because they have been published!
■ You can't get away with just reading the abstract if you want to know whether the paper is any good.
■ How to look for the smaller points (that I would normally read over) in a paper that really do make a difference in the way the research was conducted, e.g. inclusion exclusion criteria and have they accounted for who dropped out.

All you need to run this style of journal club is a quiet room, copies of the CASP tools and a group of people who have read the paper. There is no formal presentation, the discussion relies on all the people in the club not just one, and since everyone is asked at least one question there is an incentive to read the paper!

The key to a good journal club is:

▪ Everyone must read the paper.
▪ Guidance is provided to all participants about how to critically appraise.
▪ The club is supported and encouraged by senior members of staff.

5.6 Resources

There is a huge amount of information available to help with critical appraisal; this is a selection of those I have found useful.

5.6.1 Websites

Centre for Evidence Based Medicine, Oxford: this centre has been set up to improve patient care by developing and promoting evidence-based health care, and to provide support and resources, including a range of presentations and courses – http://www.cebm.net/critical_appraisal.asp

School of Health and Related Research (ScHARR), University of Sheffield: has several useful pages including a tutorial on critical appraisal and using the literature – http://www.shef.ac.uk/scharr/ir/units/critapp/index.htm; and a guide to searching the literature and a vast array of web links – http://www.shef.ac.uk/scharr/ir/netting/

Centre for Health Evidence: this site provides users' guides to evidence-based practice, including the complete set of users' guides, originally published as a series in the *Journal of the American Medical Association* – http://www.cche.net/usersguides/main.asp

Users' Guides to the Medical Literature: A Manual for Evidence Based Clinical Practice. The above articles have been enhanced and re-introduced as an on-line manual, but access requires subscription through *JAMA* – http://www.usersguides.org

Critical Appraisal Skills Programme (CASP© Milton Keynes Primary Care Trust 2002), NHS Public Health Resource Unit, Public Health Development (http://www.phru.nhs.uk/Pages/PHD/CASP.htm) provides a range of guidance on appraising research, including tools to help you appraise the following types of studies:

- Cohort
- Qualitative
- RCT
- Review
- Case-control
- Diagnostic tests
- Economic evaluation

All these tools are available on the internet for personal use and NHS organisations may reproduce or use the publication for non-commercial educational purposes provided the source is acknowledged (CASP© Milton Keynes Primary Care Trust 2002).

Scottish Intercollegiate Guidelines Network provides critical appraisal notes and checklists on their website: http://www.sign.ac.uk/methodology/checklists.html

5.6.2 Books

Iain Kinloch Crombie (1996) *The Pocket Guide to Critical Appraisal.* BMJ books, London.

Trisha Greenhalgh (2006) *How to Read a Paper. The Basics of Evidence Based Medicine*, 3rd edn. Blackwell BMJ books, London.

5.6.3 Papers

Edited highlights of *How to Read a Paper* (book listed above) have been published in the *BMJ*, all are freely available on the *BMJ* website (http://bmj.com). Use the advanced search and enter the year, volume and first page:

Greenhalgh, T. (1997) How to read a paper. The Medline database. *BMJ*, 315(7101), 180–183.

Greenhalgh, T. (1997) How to read a paper. Getting your bearings (deciding what the paper is about). *BMJ*, 315(7102), 243–246.

Greenhalgh, T. (1997) Assessing the methodological quality of published papers. *BMJ*, 315 (7103), 305–308.

Greenhalgh, T. (1997) How to read a paper. Statistics for the non-statistician. I: Different types of data need different statistical tests. *BMJ*, 315(7104), 364–366.

Greenhalgh, T. (1997) How to read a paper. Statistics for the non-statistician. II: 'Significant' relations and their pitfalls. *BMJ*, 315(7105), 422–425.

Greenhalgh, T. (1997) How to read a paper. Papers that report drug trials. *BMJ*, 315(7106), 480–483.

Greenhalgh, T. (1997) How to read a paper. Papers that report diagnostic or screening tests, *BMJ*, 315(7107), 540–543.

Greenhalgh, T. (1997) How to read a paper. Papers that tell you what things cost (economic analyses). *BMJ*, 315(7108), 596–599.

Greenhalgh, T. (1997) Papers that summarise other papers (systematic reviews and meta-analyses). *BMJ*, 315(7109), 672–675.

Greenhalgh, T., & Taylor, R. (1997) Papers that go beyond numbers (qualitative research). *BMJ*, 315(7110), 740–743.

Greenhalgh, T., & Macfarlane, F. (1997) Towards a competency grid for evidence-based practice. *J. Eval. Clin. Pract.*, 3(2), 161–165.

5.7 References

Bauchner, H., & Sharfstein, J. (2001) Failure to report ethical approval in child health research: review of published papers. *BMJ*, 323(7308), 318–319.

Bekelman, J. E., Li, Y., & Gross, C. P. (2003) Scope and impact of financial conflicts of interest in biomedical research: a systematic review. *JAMA*, 289(4), 454–465.

Gibbons, A. J. (2002) Organising a successful journal club. *BMJ Career Focus*, 325, S137a.

Gonzalez, L. S. (2003) Referees make journal clubs fun. *BMJ*, 326(11), 106.

Higgins, M., & O'Gorman, C. S. (2006) Journal club: chore or golden opportunity? *BMJ Career Focus*, 332, 212–213.

Lesser, L. I., Ebbeling, C. B., Goozner, M., Wypij, D. & Ludwig, D. S. (2007) Relationship between funding source and conclusion among nutrition-related scientific articles. *PLoS. Med.*, 4(1), e5.

6 Choosing the right research design

Following through the process so far you will have developed an initial question that you wish to answer. You will have searched the published literature for relevant information about this question and the topic area, and appraised it for quality. You may have altered your question in view of this information.

The next step is to think through how you are best going to answer this question, and what the most appropriate research design to use is. There are many excellent text books covering research design and methodology and so I do not intend to go into detail. Instead I want to provide an overview of your choices and highlight some of the thought processes you need to go through in order to make such choices.

6.1 The hierarchy of research evidence

Different research designs offer different levels of certainty about the results of the research and the idea of a hierarchy of evidence has been used widely. Traditionally, hierarchies have focused on the effectiveness of an intervention or treatment and thus the randomised control trial is regarded as the best research design for producing evidence on effectiveness, with systematic reviews of a number of randomised controlled trials at the top of the hierarchy (see Table 6.1).

However, this approach has generated controversy and much discussion about where other research designs fit into the various levels. An excellent review of the topic is given by Evans (2003), who offers a broader view of the evaluation of health care interventions. He argues that the hierarchy for the effectiveness of interventions is well placed to answer such questions as: Does the intervention work? Is it better than the usual treatment? What are the harms? However, it does not include research that can offer insight into the appropriateness and feasibility of an intervention. Clearly for an intervention to be useful it must be effective, but also acceptable to the patient and feasible to incorporate into routine health care. So Evans' proposed hierarchy may be more useful than the traditional approach if you are aiming to answer questions like:

■ What is the patient's experience?
■ What outcomes does the patient view as important?
■ Will the intervention be accepted by health care workers?
■ How can the intervention be best implemented into routine practice?

Evans' hierarchy is shown in Figure 6.1. This includes and shows the value of qualitative interpretive methods, but supports the idea that larger multi-centre trials and systematic reviews of whatever methodology will always give the most powerful evidence. As with the traditional hierarchy, case reports, opinion, and poor quality studies are ranked lowest.

Table 6.1 The traditional hierarchy of research designs which will provide the most reliable evidence for the effectiveness of treatments.

Rank	Methodology	Description
1	Systematic reviews and meta-analyses	A systematic review combines the results of a number of original studies which have been systematically searched out, judged on pre-defined inclusion criteria, and a synthesis of their results is produced. A meta-analysis is the combination of results from several independent trials to produce an overall result. A systematic review will often include a meta-analysis. Meta-analysis can be done on any selection of results but it is only regarded as level 1 evidence if combined with a systematic review.
2	Randomised controlled trials	Trial participants are randomly assigned to either a control group or a treatment group who receive a specific intervention. The aim is to control all other factors that may influence the effect of the intervention.
3	Cohort studies	Two or more groups of people who have a different exposure to a particular agent (like smoking, a vaccine, or type of surgery) are selected and then followed up to see what differences there are between the groups for specific outcomes.
4	Case-control studies	People with a particular condition (cases) are matched with people without the condition (controls), and differences are then examined in a retrospective analysis.
5	Cross-sectional studies and surveys	An examination of a sample of the population of interest at one point in time. Surveys often use a questionnaire or interview design.
6	Case reports	A report based on a single patient which can sometimes be collected together into a short series.
7	Expert opinion	A consensus from the experts in the field.
8	Anecdotal	Observations made through clinical practice which link a particular outcome with a particular condition or intervention.

	Effectiveness	Appropriateness	Feasibility
Excellent	• Systematic review • Multi-centre studies	• Systematic review • Multi-centre studies	• Systematic review • Multi-centre studies
Good	• RCT • Observational studies	• RCT • Observational studies • Interpretive studies	• RCT • Observational studies • Interpretive studies
Fair	• Uncontrolled trials with dramatic results • Before and after studies • Non-randomised controlled trials	• Descriptive studies • Focus groups	• Descriptive studies • Action research • Before and after studies • Focus groups
Poor	• Descriptive studies • Case studies • Expert opinion • Studies of poor methodological quality	• Expert opinion • Case studies • Studies of poor methodological quality	• Expert opinion • Case studies • Studies of poor methodological quality

Figure 6.1 Hierarchy of evidence: ranking of research evidence evaluating health care interventions. David Evans (2003) Hierarchy of evidence. *Journal of Clinical Nursing*, 12(1), 77–84, Blackwell Publishing Ltd.

Given this information you may feel that the only worthwhile research to carry out is a randomised controlled trial. However, randomised trials can be resource intensive and expensive to run and the problem may not be answerable using this design. Thus, it is important to think through carefully what design will best answer your question and aim to undertake the type of research that will provide the strongest evidence possible.

6.2 Types of research

There are two main types of research; quantitative and qualitative. Quantitative research involves the analysis of numerical data in order to explain a pre-defined hypothesis. The researcher aims to remain objective and control the conditions of the research. Qualitative research involves the analysis of words, pictures or objects in order to explore and describe a situation, process or experience. The researcher interprets the data as it unfolds during the collection process and the subjective nature of the process is embraced.

Behind these types of research are different philosophical assumptions and different approaches to examining the research question. It is beyond the scope of this book to examine these differences in detail but I would recommend that you explore them, and the Resources section will guide you to useful text books. Each type of research has its own advantages and disadvantages and will answer different types of question, which I will describe in the next sections. When making your decision, think about what your chosen method will allow you to find out and also what it will not allow you to explain.

6.3 Quantitative research

The main approaches within quantitative research are experimental and observational studies. These approaches test theories and produce numerical data which are statistically analysed. The intention is always to use a sample of a population and then make inferences about the whole population from the results of the smaller samples. Data can be collected prospectively or retrospectively; in other words from the start of the study forwards or searching back through previously collected information. Data can be explored within the study sample longitudinally, to study changes over time, or cross-sectionally, to observe an occurrence at one point in time only.

6.3.1 Essential elements of experimental studies

In experimental studies we are trying to establish cause and effect. We want to show that a particular intervention causes particular effects. This is the basis of the evaluation of new therapies or procedures in health care to demonstrate effectiveness. To do this we first need to compare the new therapy (applied to the intervention group) to something else, this could be no therapy at all or the therapy that is in normal use. This is applied to the control group in the experiment.

We next need to decide what piece of information will tell us the therapy is effective and decide exactly how to measure it. This is known as the *outcome*, and I have discussed this elsewhere in Chapter 7, Section 7.2.6.5.

In order to ensure that the changes in the outcome measurement are due to the experimental therapy we need to consider *bias* – the main purpose of the experimental design is to minimise bias. Firstly, the control group should be comparable to the experimental group in all ways other than the experimental treatment. This is ideally achieved through randomisation, which ensures that the unmeasured and unmeasurable characteristics are equally distributed between the groups. Randomisation means that each person entering the study has an equal chance of being assigned to either the control or the experimental group. Randomisation is achieved through using random number tables or randomisation schedule generators on the internet (see Resources section). Despite randomisation it is still important to check that both groups are comparable, so we need to collect information about any factors that could potentially alter the response to the experimental treatment.

Another source of bias is through unconscious favouring of the intervention group over the control by both the researcher and the participants. To get round this problem, *blinding* is used. Single blinding means that either the researcher measuring the outcome (the assessor) does not know which group each participant is in or the participant is unaware of the group they are in. *Double blinding* means that neither the participant nor the researcher knows which group the participant is in. A placebo is commonly used in drug trials and sometimes in other types of therapy, and is designed so that the control group think they are receiving the same treatment as the experimental group. This allows the psychological effect of simply receiving a treatment to be taken into account. In many therapy trials it is not possible to use a placebo or achieve double blinding and in this circumstance it is crucial that every effort is made to blind the assessor to the treatments, so that the measurement of the outcome that demonstrates the effectiveness of the treatment is subject to the least bias possible.

Bias can also occur if the method of measuring the outcome is difficult and prone to variation, for example blood pressure or ultrasound measurements. This variation can be minimised by taking several measurements and using the mean of the two or three measurements; this is known as *replication*.

The preceding description describes the components of the randomised controlled trial, which, as I have discussed in Section 6.1, is regarded as the best form of experiment. The absence of any of these essential elements reduces the strength of the evidence produced by the research. For example, the absence of randomisation reduces the design to what is termed a quasi-experimental design, where there is a control group but the treatment is not assigned randomly. In this case it is difficult to argue that the control is similar to the experimental group and there may be differences between the two groups that could account for any effect observed. It is always better to plan a proper experimental trial and if this is not possible you need to be able to justify why a quasi-experimental approach is to be used.

6.3.2 Observational studies

Observational studies do not include a research intervention; instead participants are monitored or observed. Observational studies explore associations between factors to establish the development of a disease or condition. Examples include studies examining smoking and cancer, where people who smoke and those who do not are compared to evaluate the effects of smoking. Often observational studies are essential since the factors involved are not amenable to randomisation. We can not randomly ask people to smoke or not to smoke, or dictate a level of compliance or predict certain complications. Such studies can provide evidence of likely causes of diseases or complications, for which treatments or preventative measures can then be sought. Observational studies include cohort, case control, and cross-sectional studies. Also categorised as observational are descriptive studies such as surveys and case studies or case series. A simple description of each is given in Table 6.1.

As with experimental studies there are important elements that must be considered in each design, particularly the minimisation of bias. Selection of the sample is particularly important since it must represent the larger population as closely as possible, and in case control studies, controls must match the cases closely. Where retrospective data are being used there will be problems with recall bias and the reliability of retrospective data. Recall bias occurs when cases (people with the disease or problem) are more likely than controls to recall the factors they think might have caused the problem or when the controls under-report exposure to possible causative factors. Anyone working in health care will understand the problems with obtaining data retrospectively; often medical notes are not complete or cannot be located, and the data reported in notes are not necessarily consistent between different patients.

In prospective studies it is important to fully follow up all the original patients recruited to the study. Loss to follow up can make the results less reliable. This is a problem for all prospective studies, including experimental studies, but is particularly relevant to cohort studies, which can often involve a large number of participants over a long period of time. A similar problem, low response rate, occurs with surveys, where the validity of the results relies on a large proportion of those being surveyed actually responding.

Sections 6.3.1 and 6.3.2 provide a synopsis of the issues to think about when using particular quantitative designs. I have intentionally kept this to a minimum as research design is a huge topic and you will certainly have to obtain more detailed information on your chosen research design in other specialised texts (see Resources section). Table 6.2 summarises the most common uses of each research design and lists the advantages and disadvantages.

6.4 Qualitative research

I came to qualitative research later in my research career. Qualitative research does suffer an image problem with researchers strongly oriented to the quantitative approach; however, this is slowly changing and the value of qualitative work is being increasingly recognised. Quantitative methods fail to provide information on the context of the studied situation, and is limited by the highly structured format and a high level of control put on the situation of study.

Qualitative research can provide a much more holistic view of the problem under investigation, including information that cannot be reduced to numbers. The approach to the data collection and design of the study is more flexible, as is the subsequent analysis and interpretation of collected

Table 6.2 The advantages and disadvantages of different quantitative research designs.

Research design	Advantages	Disadvantages
Randomised controlled trial	Provides the best form of evidence for the effectiveness of interventions. Enables the researcher to control for a variety of variables. Minimises bias. Allows determination of causality.	Needs careful planning to ensure good methodology considering randomisation, blinding, and sample size. In some cases randomisation is not ethical. Can be expensive and requires high levels of researcher input and time. Can be impractical and unfeasible if the sample sizes required are large.
Cohort study	Allows comparison of people who are 'exposed' to a particular event, procedure or risk factor, with those who are not. Can provide evidence of the factors that influence the cause or the progression of a disease. Can be useful where ethical issues prevent randomisation.	Weaker level of evidence for establishing causation. Bias is inevitably introduced due to the lack of randomisation. The cases may not be similar to the controls in important ways. Often need to be very large and have a long follow-up to allow sufficient cases of the disease of interest to occur during the study. Can be very costly to run due to the need for rigorous follow up and the large sample sizes.
Case control study	Allows comparison of patients with a particular disease or condition with those who have not got it. Efficient since they start with the cases and so the sample size can be kept to a minimum to demonstrate an association. Relatively easy to run. Cheaper than randomised controlled trials or cohort studies. No follow up issues.	Weaker level of evidence for establishing causation and association. Prone to bias due to recall, selection, missing retrospective data and use of inappropriate controls.

Table 6.2 Continued

Research design	Advantages	Disadvantages
Cross-sectional study	Allows a snap shot of a group of individuals who have a condition and comparison with those who do not. Also useful for validation and reliability studies or screening of diagnostic tools. As data are collected currently this design does not have the issues with bias in case control studies. No follow-up issues. Relatively cheap and easy to run.	Provides weak evidence of associations. Sample selection can be difficult and needs to represent the total population. The associations identified do not allow identification of the time sequence of events. So if a group of malnourished patients were compared to a group of well nourished it is likely the malnourished would be less healthy. But are they malnourished due to ill health or has poor health occurred due to poor nutrition?
Survey (type of descriptive cross-sectional study)	Can be used to explore a wide variety of issues such as prevalence, characteristics of a population or views and opinions. Provide descriptive data and generate hypotheses, guiding future research. Relatively cheap and easy to run. No follow up issues. It is feasible to use random samples for the total population of interest.	No evidence of associations or causality. Descriptive information only. Low response rates can limit applicability of results. Responders can differ to those who do not respond – volunteer bias.
Case report or case series	Provides descriptive data about a single case or several similar cases. Easy to do as part of clinical practice. Can generate hypotheses and guide future research. Can be useful to learn from very rare cases.	No evidence of associations or causality. Descriptive information only. Observation of few cases can be very misleading and due simply to chance. Contributes little to improving clinical practice.

information, allowing the researcher to evolve their view of the problem under investigation and adapt to the changing view. The qualitative approach also allows the researcher to interact with the research subjects in their own language and on their own terms. This approach gives a deeper understanding of the problems faced in health care and can help evaluate treatment in terms of appropriateness and feasibility discussed in Section 6.1.

The philosophy behind qualitative design recognises that there may be more than one world view; different researchers can interpret the same data in different ways. From the view of a quantitative researcher this is a disadvantage, but provided the underlying philosophy is explicitly recognised in the analysis, it can be an advantage to explore problems from a variety of viewpoints. Nevertheless, qualitative research cannot investigate causality and focuses on the content and value of information. Another potential disadvantage is that extensive and high level interviewing and questioning skills are required by a qualitative researcher in order to obtain consistent and reliable data from the respondents.

Since health care provision can be extremely complex a randomised controlled trial may not be able to define the parts of the whole package of care that contribute to the health improvements derived. As an example, implementing a dedicated stroke unit is an extremely complex intervention compared to using a new drug. The randomised controlled trial is ideally suited to assess the drug effectiveness using a comparison with a placebo. However, the stroke unit intervention is made up of a vast range of separate factors, some of which may contribute more than others to efficacy. Thus, there is great value in exploring complex interventions using qualitative methods to obtain a greater understanding of the content, process and benefits. This is only one example of what qualitative methods can offer the researcher, and also an example of where qualitative and quantitative methods can be used together (termed mixed methodology). There are many questions that are better answered using qualitative methods, particularly in areas where there is little knowledge and a greater understanding of the problem is needed.

There are a variety of approaches to qualitative research and these include; phenomenology, grounded theory, discourse analysis, ethnography and narrative research.

6.4.1 Phenomenology

Phenomenology is an approach that aims to explore the ways in which people conceive of and interpret the world. In this view, reality is relative and subjective (Stokes 2003). Phenomenology informs and helps the understanding of a particular phenomenon from a particular view point. An example is an investigation of the ways in which patients report their satisfaction with health care (the phenomenon). The researcher used in-depth interviews to explore the process of reflection that patients went through when asked to appraise their satisfaction with received health care (Edwards, Staniszweska & Crichton 2004). The interviews provided descriptions of a range of experiences from different patients, from which an essence of the phenomenon and a generalised statement about it could be derived. A critical aspect of phenomenology is the need for the researcher to suspend their own personal views or preconceived ideas about the phenomenon (known as bracketing), and seek to understand it through the views of the participants (Cresswell 1998). The aim of this type of inquiry is to show that although the phenomenon is experienced uniquely by each person, there exists an underlying unifying meaning of the experience that is essential and invariant for all people.

6.4.2 Grounded theory

Grounded theory is the systematic inquiry into a problem aiming to develop an overall theory based on personal experiences. The emergence of new data can alter or destroy the theory, so extensive data collection is required. As the theory emerges the researcher must constantly ensure it fits new data. An example is the exploration of the barriers to evidence-based nursing in order to develop a model of what barriers exist and how they relate to each other (Hannes et al. 2007). Hannes et al. used focus groups to collect data from nurses and reduced down the responses to five main themes that helped to formulate, what they called a 'problem tree', describing the interrelating issues.

6.4.3 Discourse analysis

Discourse analysis is a research approach that focuses on how talk and text can indicate how the world is understood. Studying conversations or written communications within a particular area can aid the understanding of people's beliefs, views and attitudes towards something. An example is the analysis of conversations between pharmacists and older patients during consultations for medication review (Salter et al. 2007). The researchers analysed in detail the transcribed conversations to identify how advice was offered and how patients received it, to establish the value of such consultations.

6.4.4 Ethnography

The ethnographic researcher will observe and collect data on a group of people within their usual setting over a prolonged period of time. Ethnography is a form of inquiry that relies particularly on participant observation, focusing on the meanings of individual's actions in a particular context. The context is important to enable a true understanding of events. For example, studying the decision-making process prior to withholding artificial administration of food and fluids involved two researchers becoming part of the health care teams at two nursing homes for seven and fourteen months (The et al. 2002). They made comprehensive notes on their observations and informal conversations; recorded formal interviews and meetings; studied medical records of the patients; and kept a diary of their own behaviour and attitudes. The latter process is vital in qualitative research and allows the researcher's own preconceptions and experiences, as well as the effect of their presence, to be taken into account in the interpretation and analysis of events, and is known as reflexivity.

6.4.5 Narrative research

Narrative research is an approach which relies on the stories that people tell. Narratives are structured by the individual telling the story and will be organised in the way they see fit. How someone tells a story reflects how they have chosen to organise their thoughts and could be seen as the basis for how they acted. The order of the narrative will reflect the meaning that the storyteller wants to get across to the researcher. In a study to explore the patients' experience of living with back pain, participants were asked to tell their own back pain story from when they first encountered such pain up to the current day (Corbett, Foster & Ong 2007). These narratives were analysed to produce themes which represented commonalities between the stories, and used to try to better understand the patients' experience of this condition.

6.5 How to choose the right research design

Matching the research approach and specific design to your defined research question is the next step in the research process. The preceding sections have provided a broad overview of the available methods you could use and you now need to consider which will provide the answers you are looking for. This is easier when your research question is clear and you may need to think through your question again at this point.

Think about the following:

- What type of evidence are you trying to produce? Are you trying to 'prove' a point (quantitative) or understand something better (qualitative)?
- What research designs have other people used to answer similar questions in a different field? Would this work for your question?
- If you need a quantitative approach, use the hierarchy of evidence as a guide and aim to produce the highest level of evidence possible.

- If you need a qualitative approach, consider carefully what type of information each method will produce and decide if this will answer your question.

Don't just think about what the most ideal method is. You also have to be practical and consider your available time, budget, skills and the people you will include in the study.

Different health care professions have historically had a greater emphasis on different approaches to research, for example nursing, occupational therapy and arts therapies use a lot of qualitative research design. Comparatively dietetics, physiotherapy, medicine and speech and language therapy tend to produce more research using quantitative designs. Thus, your professional background and training may also influence your choice of problem to research and the methods you use to examine it. You will also be influenced by those around you and the mentors and advisors you can access; you are likely to be steered towards approaches that these people are familiar with. If you are a student it is wise to use methods typically supported and used by your supervisors. Nevertheless, it is useful to be aware of these pressures and try to avoid being steered away from your research question of choice simply because you are unfamiliar with the methodology needed to examine it.

6.6 Resources

6.6.1 Quantitative research

6.6.1.1 Websites

There is an online research methods textbook at AllPsych Online, The virtual psychology classroom; Online psychology texts: Research methods: http://allpsych.com/researchmethods/researchcontents.html

6.6.1.2 Books

Pring, T. (2004) *Research Methods in Communication Disorders*, John Wiley & Sons, Chichester – this was recommended to me and described as 'the best book I have ever read in the area . . . very funny and accessible'. It is written for speech and language therapists but is suitable to help any professional.

Bowling, A. (2007) *Research Methods in Health: Investigating Health and Health Services*, 2nd edn, Open University Press, Maidenhead – a broad overview of all research methods and their use in the health care situation. The author has written several other books about research methods and measuring health.

Machin, D. & Campbell, M. J. (2005) *Design of Studies for Medical Research*, John Wiley & Sons, Chichester – a comprehensive text book on designing quantitative research.

6.6.2 Qualitative research

6.6.2.1 Books

The following are useful books explaining qualitative methodologies in more detail:

Cresswell, J. W. (1998) *Qualitative Inquiry and Research Design: Choosing Among Five Traditions*. Sage, Thousand Oaks, CA.

Cresswell, J. W. (2003) Qualitative procedures. In *Research Design: Qualitative, Quantitative and Mixed Method Approaches*, 2nd edn. Sage, London, pp. 179–207.

Green, J. & Thorogood, N. (2004) *Qualitative Methods for Health Research*. Sage, London.

Finlay, L. & Ballinger, C. (2006) *Qualitative Research for Allied Health Professionals – Challenging Choices*. John Wiley and Sons, London.

6.6.2.2 Papers

Hughes, D. H. (2004) The lived experience of loss: A phenomenological study. *American Psychiatric Nurses Association*,10(1), 24–32.

Price-Lackey, P. & Cashman, J. (1996) Jenny's story: reinventing oneself through occupation and narrative configuration. *Am. J. Occup. Ther.*, 50(4), 306–314.

Ballinger, C. & Payne, S. (2000) Discourse analysis: Principles, applications and critique. *British Journal of Occupational Therapy*, 63(12), 566–572.

Finlay, L. (1999) Applying phenomenology in research: problems, principles and practice. *British Journal of Occupational Therapy*, 69(7), 299–306.

Savage, J. (2000) Ethnography and health care. *BMJ*, 321, (7273), 1400–1402.

6.7 References

Corbett, M., Foster, N. E., & Ong, B. N. (2007) Living with low back pain – stories of hope and despair, *Soc. Sci. Med.*, 65(8), 1584–1594.

Cresswell, J. W. (1998) *Qualitative Inquiry and Research Design: Choosing Among Five Traditions*. Sage, Thousand Oaks, CA.

Edwards, C., Staniszweska, S., & Crichton, N. (2004) Investigation of the ways in which patients' reports of their satisfaction with healthcare are constructed. *Sociology of Health & Illness*, 26(2), 159–183.

Evans, D. (2003) Hierarchy of evidence: A framework for ranking evidence evaluating healthcare interventions. *J. Clin. Nurs.*, 12(1), 77–84.

Hannes, K., Vandersmissen, J., De Blaeser, L., Peeters, G., Goedhuys, J., & Aertgeerts, B. (2007) Barriers to evidence-based nursing: A focus group study. *J Adv. Nurs.*, 60(2), 162–171.

Salter, C., Holland, R., Harvey, I., & Henwood, K. (2007) 'I haven't even phoned my doctor yet.' The advice giving role of the pharmacist during consultations for medication review with patients aged 80 or more: qualitative discourse analysis, *BMJ*, 334(7603), 1101.

Stokes, P. (2003) *Philosophy – 100 Essential Thinkers*. Arcturus Publishing, London.

The, A. M., Pasman, R., Onwuteaka-Philipsen, B., Ribbe, M., & van der, W. G. (2002) Withholding the artificial administration of fluids and food from elderly patients with dementia: Ethnographic study. *BMJ*, 325(7376), 1326.

7 Writing the initial research protocol

You should now have your focused research question and a clear idea of the research methodology and study design you need to use to answer it. The next stage is to write a detailed research protocol. This is a document outlining exactly why you are doing the project, how you will carry it out, when it will get done and who is involved.

7.1 Why do I need a research protocol?

The research protocol is an essential document for all research projects whatever their size. It should be written before you launch into ethics or grant applications. The writing process will help to clarify your ideas and the details of methods you will use. It will also allow others to comment on your ideas. It can take many hours to fully develop your protocol and it should be seen as a process of evolution. Do not expect to get it right first time; get lots of comments from suitable people and expect to write several versions.

Once you have written your basic document it can then be fairly easily adapted for submission to ethics or grant giving bodies. After your research is underway the protocol will become a vital source of reference which ensures a consistent approach. Finally, when the data collection is done the protocol can be used as the basis for any written paper or report. It will also be a source of verification for regulatory bodies that may check to ensure you are running your study according the agreed protocol.

7.2 How is a protocol structured?

There is no fixed structure for protocols but the following sections outline suitable elements which will guide you: title, abstract, research question, hypothesis or aim, introduction and background, methods, research team, references, timetable, resources and budget, and appendices. Using these headings will give you a structure; however, the list is not exhaustive and may include items that are not relevant to your particular study design. While you are writing you may be unable to complete some sections initially, but this will highlight to you where you need more advice (for example in the analysis section). The draft protocol will be extremely useful to you in getting appropriate and accurate advice from others. Instead of trying to explain your problem you can simply show your advisor the protocol so far indicating which sections you are struggling with. Your advisor will then be able to provide better advice as they have all the information in front of them.

Most importantly there are no word limits for your research protocol; it can be as long as it needs to be. This is a refreshing change from writing up your work, when you will often be severely restricted to specific word limits. This document should be detailed and comprehensive.

7.2.1 Title page

The title is important; it is the first thing that is read and should indicate clearly what the project is about. The title needs to be concise, but also contains enough information to say what you are going to do. Typically titles contain the following elements:

- study design (such as randomised controlled trial, phenomenology, survey or pilot study)
- the problem or patient group (such as depression, patients with type 1 diabetes or fatigue)
- the main outcome of the research (such as patients' experience, better quality of life or improved mobility)
- intervention and comparison (if you have one, such as hydrotherapy versus land based exercises or high carbohydrate diet compared to high fat diet)

On the title page include the authors' names and affiliations, plus a date and version number for the protocol. A version number will ensure any changes you make to the protocol, especially once the research has started, can be tracked and linked to appropriate approvals, such as ethical approval.

7.2.2 Abstract

Although this is always placed at the start of the document and is the first section anyone will read you must write it last. It should be a summary of what you are going to do, why and what its value is. It is not a summary of the background information; it must include details of the methods, expected outcomes and potential value of the research. Limit yourself to 300–400 words only and write it for a very busy researcher or manager who wants to gain a brief overview of the whole study before looking at the details. Further information on writing abstracts can be found in Chapter 16, Section 16.1.

7.2.3 Research question

This bit should be easy since you already have your research question defined (see Chapter 3).

7.2.4 Hypothesis or aims

It may be appropriate, particularly for experimental research, to couch your question as a hypothesis. A hypothesis is a statement of what your experiment is attempting to demonstrate. However, in statistics we test what is called a null hypothesis, which is a statement of the situation where there is no difference or association to be found. For example:

Research question: What is the influence of a hospital environment compared to the home environment on patients' cognitive function and subsequent ability to perform activities of daily living after brain injury?

Hypothesis: Patients with brain injury will demonstrate better cognitive function and improved ability to perform activities of daily living in the home compared to the hospital environment.

Null hypothesis: There will be no difference in the cognitive function of patients with brain injury or their subsequent ability to perform activities of daily living, in the home compared to the hospital environment.

For qualitative or other exploratory research a hypothesis will not be needed but instead it might be useful to state the aims of the research. Your research question may be broken into several parts and these can be made explicit as aims. For example:

Research question: What are the factors that influence obese patients to successfully complete the lifestyle clinic weight loss programme?

Aims:

- To establish how patients experience the lifestyle clinic.
- To identify factors which promote the successful completion of the programme.
- To identify factors that result in patients leaving the programme.

7.2.5 Introduction or background

The introduction should be a summary of what research has been done so far in this field, what the gaps in the current knowledge are and how your research will add to the body of knowledge. Try to answer the following questions:

- **What does the published literature say?** Remember, this is where your critical appraisal skills (Chapter 5) are put to use, since you must evaluate each piece of research to judge how sound the information and conclusions are. You need to present an overall picture of the robust and reliable research that is available. Weak and flawed studies do not add much to the knowledge base and should generally be ignored. If you include assumptions based on flawed studies in your reasoning for undertaking your research you leave yourself open to criticism that the basis for your study is unsound. Nevertheless, weaker studies may provide some evidence for your proposed hypothesis and help you justify why your research project is needed.

- **What are the gaps in the information?** You might include here a brief mention of flawed studies to demonstrate you have a comprehensive knowledge of the literature available and recognise which papers do not inform your study and why. You can also highlight the gaps in the knowledge in your particular research area, which will lead on to the next section.

- **What will this particular piece of work add to the body of research?** The summary of the larger body of published research should lead you on to state how your research question will fit into the gaps and add to the general knowledge base.

- **Why do we need to know this?** You need to justify why your particular research idea is important and this will invariably mean showing how it will improve patient health or social care.

- **What value to patients, the health service, or your profession, will it have?** Think carefully about how your work will help patients because, ultimately, that is what we are all trying to do; yet this desire can get lost in the detail. This may include evidence that patients think this research question is important, and that the work links to government guidance, hospital targets or professional research priorities. This information will really strengthen your proposal should you need to obtain funding (more about this in Chapter 9).

7.2.6 Methodology or methods

In this section you explain exactly how you will carry out the research and you may need to include the following subheadings. The exact headings required will vary depending on your study design, but many of these headings are applicable for all research; qualitative and quantitative.

7.2.6.1 Study design

State the design of your study. Is it prospective or retrospective? Is it observational or experimental? Is it controlled and randomised? What are the philosophical assumptions underlying the research? What strategies of inquiry are to be used (phenomenology, grounded theory etc)? See Chapter 6 for more detail.

7.2.6.2 Location

Where will you carry out this research? Not only will you state here your organisation and geographical location but also think about which room you can use and the amount of space you need. Writing this section may result in a list of clarifications to make before the research can commence. For example; Who do you need to ask? Who else uses the room? Do you need to share and co-ordinate with others? Will you need to go to the patient's own home? Do you need to book rooms for interviews or focus groups?

7.2.6.3 Subjects

Who will you include in your study? What are your specific inclusion and exclusion criteria? How many people will you include and how have you arrived at this figure? In quantitative studies you will usually need to justify recruitment figures with a power calculation (see Chapter 8, Section 8.2.3 for details). In qualitative work you will need to explain why you have decided on the recruitment figure and what strategies you have for increasing data collection should you need to.

7.2.6.4 Recruitment

Describe how you will locate and recruit your subjects (see Chapter 13 for information on recruitment), and demonstrate that you are likely to meet your recruitment target within the proposed time span. For example, if you see on average 100 patients from the group you are interested in each year, and you need to recruit 50 to your study, you need to estimate how long it will take to recruit this number. DO NOT overestimate how many people you can recruit; this is a very common and easy error to make (I've made it several times being quite optimistic!). For even the easiest study not everyone will want to take part; for an onerous protocol or a sensitive topic maybe only 10% of screened patients will take part. You have exclusion criteria and so there will be people who are unsuitable to take part; check this carefully with your proposed pool of potential participants, you may be surprised how many people are excluded. Finally, always allow for some people to drop out. 20% is a reasonable drop out figure for most research, but studies including elderly or critical care patients may be higher. Each patient group will differ so it is a good idea to ask someone who has done research in your area.

7.2.6.5 Outcomes

Outcomes are the changes and effects that happen as a result of the intervention you are testing or the specific information and knowledge gained as a result of your investigation. You need to identify what outcomes you are expecting and looking for.

In quantitative research you will need to identify your most important outcome; the one most pertinent to your research question. This is termed the 'primary outcome' and you will use this outcome to calculate how many patients to include in your study (using a power calculation – see Chapter 8, Section 8.2.3). You may also list other outcomes of interest which you will be examining and these are termed 'secondary outcomes'.

An example of outcomes from a quantitative research hypothesis:

▪ Patients with brain injury will demonstrate better cognitive function and improved ability to perform activities of daily living in the home compared to the hospital environment.

The primary outcome will be the ability of the patient to perform activities of daily living and the secondary outcome will be a measure of cognitive function.

7.2.6.6 Measuring your outcomes

Now you have identified WHAT you are going to measure you must decide and justify HOW you are going to measure it. For example there are several ways to measure ability in activities of daily living and cognitive function. You need to think about what measures are reliable and valid in the patient group you are studying, and what is practical with the resources you have. It is very important to consider the validity of the measurement and its reliability in the situation where you will be using it. If there are questions about the validity or reliability of the outcome measure, your whole research project could be futile. If there is no valid and reliable tool to measure your chosen outcome you need to think again or first develop a suitable tool and demonstrate its validity and reliability. Also think carefully about the practicalities: What equipment do you require? Who will do the measurements? Will you need to pay for the test (perhaps you need blood analysis done)? How long will the measurement take? Do you need to take samples, and if so, where can they be stored? Describe in detail how you will carry out your measurement and include copies of questionnaires or measurement procedures in appendices. The Resource section contains further information about developing your own questionnaire.

In qualitative research your outcomes of interest will relate to your study aims but will be less defined. The nature of qualitative research is one of exploration without preconceived notions of what you will find, thus the definition of expected outcomes is less important. Nevertheless, in this section you can describe in more detail the process of obtaining the information, such as interview and focus group guides, document or audio-visual material you will use, protocols for observation and the use of diaries or journals.

An example of outcomes in a qualitative research question:

■ What are the factors that influence obese patients to successfully complete the lifestyle clinic weight loss programme?

Aims:

- To establish how patients experience the lifestyle clinic.
- To identify factors which promote the successful completion of the programme.
- To identify factors that result in patients leaving the programme.

The aims outline the broad areas of interest which will guide initial questioning but the specific outcomes are unknown until the research is complete.

7.2.6.7 Ethical considerations

All research requires ethical approval and the main job of the ethics committee is to weigh up whether the risks and burdens placed on the participants are not unduly onerous and are balanced by the benefits. In the ethics application you will be asked for specific information about numerous aspects of your research (covered in detail in Chapter 10), but in this section of the protocol it is useful to consider the broad issues at stake. Think about how you will recruit and include patients within an ethical framework. Are there any difficult ethical issues to consider, for example studying children or adults with dementia? What are the main risks and burdens for your participants? How will you maintain confidentiality and data protection? For studies with interventions consider which criteria will lead to withdrawal of patients and how you will record and report adverse events.

7.2.6.8 Study plan

In this section you need to describe in detail exactly how the research will be carried out. Take the reader through the process step by step explaining what you will do and what the patient will need to do. Start from when you recruit the person and obtain informed consent and go through to the end of the study. Include how you plan to randomise (if relevant), what will be done at each assessment or interview, the frequency of assessments or interviews, and what happens at the end of the study. Someone else should be able to pick up the information and repeat the work. A flow diagram of the study process can be valuable for studies with more than two visits.

7.2.6.9 Plan of analysis

For both qualitative and quantitative research this is an extremely important section to think through at this early stage. This is the plan you will use for the future analysis of the data and it will help to make sure you collect the appropriate information.

In quantitative research this plan needs to be clearly defined (known as *a priori* analysis) with the purpose of testing each specified hypothesis. An analysis that you decide to do later which is outside the original plan (known as *post hoc* analysis), perhaps once you have looked at your data, will not bear the same weight as the planned analysis. Post hoc analyses are regarded as hypothesis *generating* whereas a priori analyses are hypothesis *testing*. This means the results from post hoc analyses ideally need to be further tested by another trial that is specifically set up to test that hypothesis. You need to plan what analysis is required to test your stated hypotheses and any other analysis that you predict you will need to explain your results or control for confounding factors.

In my experience a lot of novice researchers panic or just ignore this section and hope they think of something by the time they have collected the data. This is an easy trap to fall into since most people will have little idea of how to think through the analysis if they have never done it before. Therefore, it is vital that you get advice from a more experienced researcher or a statistician. The Resources sections in this chapter and Chapter 8 contain suggested sources of information that may help. In Chapter 8 I look in more detail at planning your statistical analysis. Some of the broad issues you need to include in this section are the method of data analysis, the proposed comparisons or investigations of relationships, the programs to be used for data analysis and who is going to do the analysis.

With qualitative research you must also describe how you intend to approach your analysis. This is less prescriptive than quantitative analysis but there are specific steps you should consider, then describe how you will approach each step. These include: organising and preparing your data for analysis, conducting the preliminary analysis to gain a general sense of the data, conducting more detailed analysis including coding, describing the data by producing themes, and finally how you will represent and interpret the data (Cresswell 2003). Your analysis will be driven by the methodology you have chosen to use in your study and the underpinning philosophical assumptions.

7.2.7 *The research team*

In this section you need to demonstrate why you are the right person or team to do this research. Writing this section will help you clarify each team member's role in the project and identify where you may need another's expertise. This section is also crucial if you are going to apply for grant funding; you will need to convince the funder that your team will deliver high quality research within the agreed time frame. This section will allow you to show that you have the right mix of expertise in your team and enough manpower to make sure the work gets done.

7.2.8 *References*

Your work should always be supported by referencing published literature. If you make firm statements you need to be able to back them up with evidence. If you do not have the evidence you need to make this clear in your writing. Thus, at the end of any scientific document you will be expected to include a list of references you have used. In your protocol this should be comprehensive and extensive.

Referencing requires you to make 'in-text citations', which are short references to the full information, and then a reference list at the end of your document containing all the information required to find each specific document that you have cited. The in-text citation is either the author name and date of publication (Hickson, 2007) or simply a number (1) which leads you to the full information in the reference list.

In your protocol, it does not matter what style you use to cite your references but do make sure you use one style consistently. I would recommend the Harvard style as this means you include the author and date in the text and then list the references in alphabetical order. Including the author in the text makes it easier to see what references you have used without constantly having to refer to the list at the end and it is easy to locate whether you have already cited a particular reference. This book is referenced in Harvard style. The other commonly used style is Vancouver, which requires each reference to be numbered in the text and then listed in cited order. There are slight differences in how the information in the reference list are ordered and presented between the two styles. To find details of how to reference in either Harvard or Vancouver either ask in your library or search the internet using 'Harvard' or 'Vancouver' and 'reference' as search terms.

Ultimately which style you use is really a matter of personal preference, so find a style that you like or find out if your institution requires you to use a certain style. When you come to submitting grant applications and journal articles, the style of referencing may well be specified but if you use reference management software (see Section 4.2) changing the style is a matter of clicking a few buttons.

Do reference your work as you go along – do not leave it all to the end. I have made this mistake and can confirm that it is extremely frustrating to know you have read a paper supporting a particular point but simply can't recall the author or remember where you have put the paper! It is also a tedious and boring job to do it all at the end; it is much better to cite as you write, and make sure the full reference information is added to your reference list or into your reference management software as you go along.

7.2.9 Timetable

When planning your research project you need to think through how long it is all going to take. There are various stages in the research process (as this book aims to illustrate) and you need to consider each stage and how long it will take. If this is the first time you have planned research this is difficult to do, so do ask experienced folk and try not to underestimate.

An example of a timetable displayed as a gantt chart is given in Figure 7.1. You can display your timetable in any format you prefer, for example as a list or table specifying dates or number of months. The idea is to give a broad estimate of how long the whole project will take and the intermediate milestones along the way. Everyone knows that these time spans may not be met precisely since unforeseen problems can occur, but you need to give the most realistic estimate you can.

	Month											
	1	2	3	4	5	6	7	8	9	10	11	12
Obtain ethics	▓	▓	▓									
Design data collection forms and data spread sheet and other preparation work	▓	▓										
Commencement of data collection and recruitment				▓	▓	▓	▓					
Assessment 2 in data collection phase						▓	▓	▓				
Data entry & checking								▓	▓			
Data analysis										▓		
Write report											▓	▓

Figure 7.1 Gantt chart to demonstrate a time plan for a research project.

7.2.10 Resources and budget

Any research will invariably impact on resources in some way, and often is impossible to do without a specific budget. When you are planning research you will have to decide whether it can be achieved within current resources or whether you need to apply for funding. How to obtain research funding is covered in Chapter 9.

Remember this is your protocol and not a grant application, so don't worry too much about getting precise quotes yet. The purpose of this section is to allow you to think through what resources you need and roughly what they will cost, and allow you to consider the best way to support them. When developing a budget for a research project you need to carefully balance what you really need to make the research happen with how much you think you can ask for in grant funding. In the protocol at this stage it is better to include everything; you can then whittle this down to suit a particular grant application should you need to.

It is amazing what can be achieved with tiny amounts of money or no money at all when there is a combined determination to get the work done. This is particularly true of small pilot projects that novice researchers are most likely to be planning. If you, your research team, your manager and organisation want the work done, you will almost certainly find a way. For larger studies there is no doubt funding will be required and this section will be the first step in defining exactly what you need. The following sub-sections list the items you need to consider under resources.

7.2.10.1 Personnel

Can this research be done within your team's current workload or do you need to employ a person to support your workload or do the research? How much will that cost?

7.2.10.2 Equipment, materials and supplies

List exactly what equipment or supplies you need and how much they will cost. Remember to think about office supplies, postage and photocopying, as well as the equipment costs or costs of blood or sample analysis.

7.2.10.3 Travel expenses

You may need to consider reimbursing travel expenses or compensating for time, particularly if you are using healthy volunteers. For patients you must consider how they will attend any appointments and you may need to pay their costs. Don't forget your own travel too; do you need to go out and visit patients at home? Do you need to run focus groups away from your place of work? You may also like to include travel costs to a conference to present your results.

7.2.10.4 Other expenses

This could include registration to attend conferences to present your results, the costs of consultancy work (such as a statisticians' fees for doing the analysis or providing advice), the costs of hiring venues for group work or interviews, recruitment costs if you need to advertise your research post, administrative support and so on.

7.2.11 Appendices

It is entirely appropriate to include appendices in your protocol for future reference. It will be particularly useful to include specific questionnaires you plan to use in your research, measurement protocols, quotes for equipment, job descriptions of potential posts should the research be funded and any other supporting information.

7.3 Peer review of your protocol

The research governance framework states that all research should undergo peer review at some stage to ensure robust and rigorous methodology (more detail on governance is given in Chapter 2). Any studies being submitted for funding will usually be peer reviewed for the funding body. However, smaller projects, to be done within work time will not automatically enter such a process. Your place of work may have a system of peer review for internal studies, or you may wish to submit your proposal to an experienced researcher, unconnected with your study, for an objective review. Your professional organisation may be able to help with finding a suitable person.

Peer review at this stage is extremely valuable; you will get useful comments on the design and rationale for your study, hopefully any particular problems or flaws will be highlighted, and it may help you clarify areas of uncertainty. What a peer reviewer does not want to do is spend time correcting basic grammar, spelling and sentence structure; they are interested in the intellectual content. Thus, if someone kindly agrees to read your work make sure you proof read it carefully first and make sure it is presented in a format that is agreeable to the reviewer. So ask if they would prefer an electronic or paper copy; you may prefer corrections in electronic format but your reviewer may want to do it on paper.

7.4 Resources

7.4.1 Websites

The Leeds Teaching Hospitals NHS Trust, R & D Homepage has guidance on how to prepare research proposals, including instructions on writing the protocol and a useful series of questions to ask yourself (focus is on quantitative methods): http://www.leedsteachinghospitals.com/sites/research_and_development/

Statistical Services Centre, Reading University provides a series of guides to be found at www.reading.ac.uk/ssc/publications/guides.html including *Writing Research Protocols – A Statistical Perspective.*

Your own local R & D office or Research and Development Support Unit (RDSU) may also offer advice or web resources, and access to statistical advice.

7.4.2 Papers

Three good papers on developing your own questionnaire:

Boynton, P. M. & Greenhalgh, T. (2004) Selecting, designing, and developing your questionnaire. *BMJ*, 328(7451), 1312–1315.
Boynton, P. M. (2004) Administering, analysing, and reporting your questionnaire. *BMJ*, 328(7452), 1372–1375.
Boynton, P. M., Wood, G. W., & Greenhalgh, T. (2004) Reaching beyond the white middle classes. *BMJ*, 328(7453), 1433–1436.

7.4.3 Books

Oppenheimer, N. (1992) *Questionnaire Design, Interviewing and Attitude Measurement.* Continuum, London – this is a detailed introduction into the use of questionnaires and interviewing.

7.5 Reference

Cresswell, J. W. (2003) Qualitative procedures. In *Research Design: Qualitative, Quantitative and Mixed Method Approaches*, 2nd edn. Sage, London, pp. 179–207.

8 Getting started with statistics

Statistics can be daunting and I have observed when helping novice researchers that statistics tend to induce two states: fear and boredom. I want to start by saying I have been there, felt that and have struggled enormously getting to grips with statistics. On one hand I feel far from qualified to advise people on this subject. Nevertheless, after my own struggles with statistics I do have empathy with those of you who share this difficulty. In this chapter I have endeavoured to outline the things you need to think about and gain more knowledge on. I can also confirm that it is not impossible and it can be interesting too, once you get to grips with the basics and stop panicking!

I would strongly recommend buying at least one good statistics book so you always have a text to refer to if things are not making sense. There are numerous excellent texts which will help you and I have provided a list of those books and other resources that I have found helpful at the end of the chapter. In addition, use every opportunity to gain a greater understanding of statistics. For example, if you attend a journal club, make it a mission to look up and fully comprehend the statistics on all the papers you appraise.

8.1 Back to basics

Before going any further I want to stop and explain some statistical terminology. Understanding the plethora of terms is half the battle in overcoming a fear of statistics. As the title states, this section takes you right back to basic maths; some readers will find this a helpful starter, for many this will be valuable revision but some may like to skip through to Section 8.2. Before you decide to skip on why don't you test yourself using the 'test questions' at the start of each section? These questions summarise what each section will tell you and enable you to find out what you really know!

8.1.1 Populations and samples

Test question: Give some examples of populations and samples.

The purpose of statistical analysis in health and social research is to use information about a sample of individuals to make inferences about the wider population. A sample is a selected group from the population of interest. Generally we are talking about people but it can be a sample of anything. For example, a study about A & E service provision may use a sample of 50 hospitals from the total 'population' of NHS Hospitals in the UK. This, you may be thinking, is obvious but it is always important to remember the underlying principles when interpreting and carrying out analyses.

8.1.2 Probability

Test question: Explain probability and why is it an important concept in statistics?

The probability of an event happening is the proportion of times the event would occur if we repeated the experiment a large number of times. This is usually expressed as a percentage or a decimal, for example, the probability of throwing 1 when tossing a dice is 1/6, 17% or 0.17. A probability of 0 means there is no chance of that event happening (probability of throwing 7), and a probability of 1 means a particular event will always happen (probability of throwing 1, 2, 3, 4, 5, or 6). You need to understand probability since this is the basis of inferential statistics.

8.1.2.1 p values

When you come to analyse data you are no doubt expecting to produce some p values; p stands for probability, and is telling you the probability of the hypothesis you are testing occurring by chance alone. As Altman (1999) states in his statistical textbook, 'Statistical analysis allows us to put limits on our uncertainty, but not to prove anything'. Statistics is all about probability.

8.1.3 Types of data

Test questions: What is the difference between continuous and discrete data? What is the difference between ordinal and nominal data? Give examples of each type.

There are various different types of data and each is analysed using different methods. Identifying which type of data you will produce in your study is the first step in planning how you will analyse it.

8.1.3.1 Numerical data

Continuous data are generally acquired using some sort of measurement and are not limited to a fixed set of values. Examples include age, weight, height, distance travelled for health care or blood sugar level. In each case, any value is possible between the biological norms, so for humans you could get values of age between 0 and say 115 years, and the precision of the measurement depends on the requirements of the particular study (whether it is in days, months or years).

Discrete data can take a value from a finite set of possible values. They are often analysed as continuous but sometimes may be better analysed using other methods. Examples include number of appointments, number of children, age at last birthday or shoe size. It is not possible to have half an appointment or 0.3 of a child and this is what distinguishes this type of data from continuous.

8.1.3.2 Categorical data

Categorical data is where the observation made can only be one option, in other words values are categorised into two or more groups. There are two main types of categorical data: ordinal and nominal. Ordinal data have a meaningful order, such as a 5 point pain scale or social class. It is important to note that you cannot assume the interval between each ordered category is the same (i.e. someone scoring 4 on a pain scale does not necessarily have twice as much pain as someone scoring 2) and this makes ordinal data different to discrete numerical data. Nominal data have no order and examples include ethnicity or blood group. Nominal data also include a special case: binary or dichotomous data, which have only two possible categories such as gender, disease or no disease and in-patient or out-patient.

8.1.4 Describing your data

There are several terms you will come across regularly when reading quantitative research papers and you will need to be able to use this terminology when you come to describing your own data. You are likely to have heard of many of the following terms but perhaps you can't actually define them. As before test yourself as you go through this section and see how much you do know or where you need more revision.

8.1.4.1 Central tendency or average

Test question: What are the three ways to describe the average value of a set of data and how do you calculate them?

There are three ways to describe the average of a set of data and which you use depends on the type of data you have. The three ways are mean, median and mode. The mean is the sum of all the observations in the data set divided by the number of observations, and this is the value usually referred to when people talk about the 'average'. The median is the middle observation when they are listed in order of increasing size. If you have an even number of observations you will have two 'middle' values and in this case you would take the mean of these two values to calculate the median. Finally the mode is the most frequently observed value in any given set of data. This is the least used of the three types of 'averages' but can be useful for discrete data.

8.1.4.2 Variation in the data

Test question: What measures of variation are there and how would you describe them?

There are three main ways to describe the variation seen in any given set of data and again which you use will depend on the data. The three ways are the range, the inter-quartile range and the standard deviation. The range is simply the maximum and minimum values. This represents the total spread of the data but tells you little about how each individual value varies from the others. This makes the range less useful but it is sometimes of value to quote it if you wish to describe the total spread of the data.

The inter-quartile range (IQR) includes the values between which the middle 50% of the data lie, or put another way are the values at the 25% and 75% percentiles. This means the values below which 25% and 75% of the data lie. The median is at the 50th centile since half the data lie below and half above this value. The inter-quartile range is useful since it describes the middle bulk of the data and excludes the increasingly extreme outlying values. A larger difference between these two values illustrates the greater variation in the data and this measure of variation is commonly used with the median.

The standard deviation (SD, sd, s, or σ) is calculated using a specific formula and provides a single figure to show the amount of variation within a set of data. A larger standard deviation equates to more variation within the set of data.

8.1.4.3 Data distributions

Test question: What kind of distributions are there and what type of average and measure of variation is most appropriate to use with these distributions?

You may well now be wondering how you decide which of these 'averages' or 'measures of variation' you should choose to use. It all pivots on the distribution of your data. Figure 8.1 shows histograms illustrating three main types of data distribution in a pure form. Obviously clinical data will never be this pure and your distribution will approximate to one or other of these types. There are several ways to find out how your data are distributed but one of the easiest is to plot a histogram and look at it. Does it look roughly normal or is it more skewed one way or the other? Figure 8.2 gives an example of a histogram plotted for a group of 134 patients aged over 50 years. If you look at the horizontal axis you will see each column covers a range of 2.5 years, thus this diagram tells you that three patients

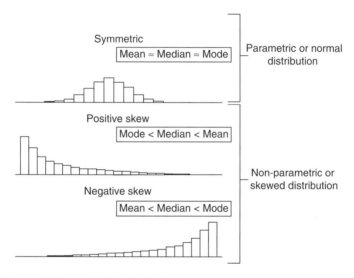

Figure 8.1 Three main types of data distribution.

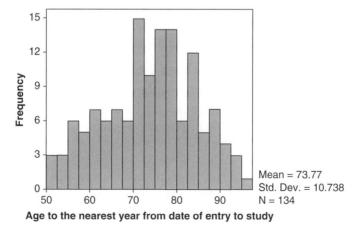

Figure 8.2 Histogram showing the age distribution in a study looking at adults over 50 years.

were aged between 50 and 52.5 years and that one was aged between 95 and 97.5 years. This histogram shows an approximately normal distribution. Histograms are very easily generated on computer statistical software so don't worry about creating such diagrams.

These distribution types are described as either normal (parametric) or skewed (non-parametric). If you read more about statistics you find several other distributions described but I am sticking to the basics here and for more detail you will need to turn to a specialist source. Looking again at Figure 8.1 will show you that the values of the different types of averages vary depending on the distribution of the data. For normal data all averages will be similar but for skewed data there are considerable differences between the mean, median and mode. For normal data the best measure to use is the mean since every value contributes to the calculation of the mean. For skewed data the best description of the central tendency is the median. The best descriptors of the amount of variation are the inter-quartile range for skewed data and standard deviation for normal data.

8.1.5 Using your data to answer your research question

We have now covered the basics for describing your data and I will move on to look at analysis. The purpose of descriptive statistics is to describe the characteristics of the study sample and you can then see how the sample fits with the general population of interest. However, to test hypotheses you need to use what are termed *inferential* statistics; put simply you are using a small sample to make inferences or draw conclusions about a larger population. Do not panic about carrying out such calculations; at this stage it is far more important to understand the principles involved and the terminology used. Actually carrying out the analysis will come later.

8.1.5.1 Hypothesis testing

Test questions: What is a null hypothesis? What does a p value of 0.05 mean?

As described earlier (see Chapter 7, Section 7.2.4), when you set up a study you have a research question which can also be phrased as a statement or hypothesis. This can then be re-phrased as a NULL hypothesis (H_0), and an example is given in Section 7.2.4. In using statistics we are trying to show the likelihood that the null hypothesis is true. Once you have defined your null hypothesis you test it using the appropriate statistical test and calculate a p value (remember p = probability). This tells you the probability of your study yielding its findings if the null hypothesis is true; or how likely were you to get these results through chance alone. For example, put simply, if

Table 8.1 A comparison of the total number of cases of antibiotic associated diarrhoea in each study group.

Diarrhoea	Probiotic (N = 57)	Control (N = 56)	p value
Yes	7 (12%)	19 (34%)	0.007
No	50 (88%)	37 (66%)	

you obtain a p value of 0.05 this means there is 5% chance that the null hypothesis is true or 95% chance it is wrong.

Table 8.1 shows some data from a published study (Hickson et al. 2007). The null hypothesis being tested here is, 'treatment with a probiotic drink will not reduce the incidence of antibiotic associated diarrhoea compared to a placebo'. The interpretation of these results is that there is a tiny (0.7%) chance of finding these results if the null hypothesis were true, therefore, it is most likely to be false and we can accept the positive hypothesis that probiotic drinks do reduce the incidence of antibiotic associated diarrhoea.

8.1.5.2 Confidence intervals

Test question: Describe a confidence interval and explain what it is telling you.

In your research you are looking at a sample but are really interested in the wider population. A confidence interval (CI) calculates two values from your sample data between which your population value is likely to fall. A narrow confidence interval (the two values are close together) indicates that the sample estimate is relatively precise but a wide interval means you can be less certain about the unknown population value.

Confidence intervals are usually shown as 95% confidence intervals although it is possible to calculate any percent value. 95% is deemed suitable for most health care research and it is almost always what you will see in papers. The 95% refers to the probability that the range shown will contain the true population value. So for a 95% confidence interval you can be 95% sure that your true population value will fall within the given range.

From the data presented in Table 8.1 the difference in the rates of diarrhoea in the two groups is 22%, and the 95% confidence interval for this difference is 7% to 37%. This means that in our small sample the reduction in diarrhoea is 22%, but in the wider population we can only estimate it to be somewhere between 7% and 37%. This is a fairly wide range and indicates that the study result (22%) is not very precise and perhaps a larger study is needed.

8.1.5.3 Choosing the right test

Test questions: List three tests that are suitable to use with normally distributed data and three with non-parametric distributed data. Explain in what circumstances you would use each test. What tests are suitable for use with categorical data? What are paired and independent data?

Another reason for establishing the distribution of the data is to help you decide how best to analyse it. Parametric data are analysed using one set of statistical tests which rely on the assumption that the data are normally distributed, and if they are not the test is not valid. For skewed data a different set of statistical tests are used which make no assumptions about the data. Table 8.2 shows the common statistical tests to use for data from different distributions. You should now be clear about what are continuous data and about the difference between parametric and non-parametric distributions. To fully interpret this table you also need to understand sample structure. This depends on the design of your research and how you have chosen to organise the comparative data collection. Paired, or related, data mean the two measures you are comparing are related in some way, usually because they come from the same group of people. Independent, or unrelated, data mean the two measures you are comparing are completely separate and not related, generally because you are comparing two separate groups of people. The latter is the classic randomised controlled trial, where one groups acts as the control and the other group receives an intervention. In some study designs you need more than two groups and in this case you will need to use different tests again.

Categorical data are analysed with different tests and the most common ones you will come across are shown in Table 8.3. You still need to decide

Table 8.2 Common statistical tests in use to compare two or more groups with continuous data from different distributions.

Sample structure	Parametric	Non-parametric
Two related/paired groups	Paired t test	Wilcoxon matched pairs signed rank sum
Two independent/unrelated groups	Two sample t test	Mann–Whitney U test
More than two groups	ANOVA	Kruskal–Wallis test

Table 8.3 The common statistical tests used to compare groups of categorical data.

Sample structure	Large sample	Small sample
Related/paired	McNemar's test	Binomial based
Independent/unrelated	Chi-squared test	Fisher's exact test

whether your data are paired or independent. The choice between the tests for large or small samples will be made when you do the analysis. At this stage you just need to be aware that you will use one or the other.

8.1.6 *Exploring relationships*

Your research may not involve making comparisons between groups and may instead be looking at exploring relationships between one or more variables. In this section I introduce some more terminology and describe statistical techniques to do this.

8.1.6.1 Looking for associations between two variables

Test questions: What technique is used to explore associations between two variables? What does the r value mean?

If you need to explore the degree of linear association between two sets of variables you will need to use *correlation*. For example, you may wish to know whether an increase in body weight relates to blood pressure increase. The analysis produces a coefficient (r), which lies between -1 and $+1$, and an exact linear relationship between two variables (such as weight and blood pressure) results in either $r = +1$ or -1. A coefficient of $+1$ means there is a positive relationship (if you do a scatter plot and mark in the line of best fit, the line goes up); higher values of one variable lead to higher values of the other. A coefficient of -1 means the relationship is negative (the line goes down); higher values of one variable lead to lower values of the other. A coefficient of zero means there is no relationship between the two variables.

In essence the correlation coefficient is a measure of the scatter of the points around an underlying linear trend; the greater the spread of the points the lower the correlation and the closer r will be to 0. As a rule of thumb to assess the degree of association the following is helpful (Altman 1999):

▨ $r = 0-0.25$ little/no relationship
▨ $r = 0.25-0.5$ fair degree
▨ $r = 0.5-0.75$ moderate/good
▨ $r = 0.75-1.0$ very good/excellent

It is extremely important to remember that a close association between two variables does not imply that one variable causes the other. In the previous example of weight and blood pressure further research has shown that there is a causal link and obesity does increase blood pressure. However, there are many other examples of associations which have no causal link but instead there is a factor common to both variables. For example, heart attacks and ice cream sales are negatively correlated (as ice cream sales go up, heart attack rates fall) but this does not mean ice cream protects against heart attacks, just that we buy more ice cream in the summer and there are fewer heart attacks at this time of year.

As with other statistical techniques there are various ways to test for correlation depending on the type and distribution of your data (Pearson's and Spearman's correlation coefficients) and whether a third influencing factor may be involved (partial correlation coefficient). You will need to study an appropriate text book to learn how to use these techniques correctly.

8.1.6.2 Describing relationships between variables

Test questions: What method is used to describe relationships between two or more variables? What is the result you get from a regression analysis?

Correlation simply indicates the strength of the association between two variables but it does not tell us how the variables are related or how one variable may predict the other. To obtain this type of information, *regression analysis* is required. Regression analysis should only be attempted with help from a statistician or researcher experienced in using these techniques. It is not straightforward and can be easy to get wrong.

8.1.7 Back to basics summary

I have outlined in the previous sections some of the basic information you need to understand and use statistics for health care research. Of course there is much more to learn but I hope this brief jargon busting overview will help give you confidence to tackle learning more about statistics as you go along. This section does not replace a good statistics text book written by a statistician. The underlying mathematics behind the statistical tests may remain a mystery but you can still learn to use, understand and interpret statistics.

8.2 Use of statistics throughout the research process

Having provided a summary of basic statistical terms and tests I now want to return back to the development of your research protocol. There are several phases throughout the research process that require the use of statistics and these should be thought through at an early stage and described in your protocol.

8.2.1 Design of the study

The design of your study (covered in Chapter 6) will dictate the type of analysis you will need to use. Think through whether you want to make comparisons, explore relationships or simply describe your population. For experimental studies you will need to think about blinding, bias and how you will assign patients to different groups (randomisation).

8.2.2 Representative sampling

It is important, particularly in observational studies, to make sure your sample is as similar as possible to the larger population it represents. Ideally, this would be done by randomly sampling the entire population, and for some large national surveys this is indeed what is attempted. However, in general, you will obtain your sample from the population available to you; patients that attend your out-patient clinic; the critical care patients that go through your intensive care unit; or the staff working in your local area. It is important that when you come to report your study you can describe in detail your study group; you must therefore consider what variables you need to measure or observe in order to describe the characteristics of the sample adequately. If you are involved in larger studies where you need to randomly select patients for inclusion you will need to get further advice from a statistician or epidemiologist.

8.2.3 Determining sample size

In all quantitative studies you need to decide at the start the size of your study sample. There are conflicting pressures in this decision; the larger the study sample the longer and more expensive the study will be, but a smaller sample size makes it harder to find a conclusive answer. In order to make this decision more objective you are required to do a power calculation. Essentially a power calculation estimates how big the sample needs to be in order to be sure of detecting whether your null hypothesis is true. So if you fail to disprove your null hypothesis you will be sure this is because there is nothing to find, not just because your sample size is too small. Power calculations will vary depending on your study design, but I have provided an example of the information you need for the comparison of two groups using a continuous variable. You need four items of information to do this power calculation:

■ The standard deviation of the variable of interest in each study group (the usual amount of variability of this measurement). This can be obtained from previous research in similar groups or a pilot study.

▪ The effect size – this is the smallest clinically relevant difference between the two groups that you would hope to find, and requires your clinical judgement to estimate how big an effect is clinically interesting.
▪ The significance level (α) – this is the probability of rejecting the null hypothesis when in fact it is true, and is almost always set at 0.05 or 5%, but can be set lower at 0.01 (1%).
▪ The power (β) – this is the probability that you will detect a difference if there is one to find (correctly rejecting the null hypothesis) and so this is set high, usually somewhere between 0.80 and 0.95 (80% to 95%).

These four figures will fit into a formula and produce an estimate of the number of subjects needed. In general the higher the power and lower the significance level the larger the study population will be. Also the more variation (larger sd) and the smaller the effect size, the larger the study population will need to be. There are sample size calculators on the internet (see the Resources section) and if you are certain about the figures you need and the appropriate calculation to use, they can be a convenient way to do your calculation. However, they can be confusing so I would advise obtaining the help of an experienced researcher or a statistician.

The description of the power calculation would read something like this:

A power calculation assuming a power of 90%, $\alpha = 0.05$, sd = 150 kcal and to detect a difference of 100 kcal between the two groups, resulted in an estimated sample size of 50 people in each group.

8.2.4 Analysing the data

It is important to decide what your plan of analysis will be before you start the project as I discussed in Section 7.2.6.9. You will need to specify the method of data analysis, which means deciding what type of data you will generate and what tests you may need to use. At this stage you will not be able to say how the data are distributed and thus it is common to state the two alternative tests you could use. You must specify the proposed comparisons or investigations of relationships, and ideally you will state the null hypotheses you will be testing. You may also predict that a particular subgroup requires further testing and you must state what tests are planned. Remember you are outlining your a priori analysis and any analysis not described in your protocol is regarded as post hoc and carries less weight. You should also list what computer software you will use to do the analysis and who will carry it out. I will discuss these issues further in Chapter 14.

8.3 Resources

8.3.1 Useful books

Altman, D. (1991) *Practical Statistics for Medical Research*, Chapman & Hall, London – this is my bible for statistics. It is very comprehensive and gives excellent examples to aid understanding. It does include sections on the mathematics behind analyses but the author recognises that not everyone will want to read them!

Siegel, S. & Castellan, N. J. (1998) *Nonparametric Statistics for the Behavioral Sciences*, 2nd edn, McGraw-Hill, London – someone else's bible. The text goes from completely basic to quite high level in an accessible style.

Dytham, C. (2003) *Choosing and Using Statistics, A Biologists Guide*, 2nd edn, Blackwell Science, Oxford – recommended as an easy read, written from the point of view of biologists not statisticians.

Swinscow, T. D. V. & Campbell, M. J. (2002) *Statistics at Square One*, 10th edn, BMJ Books, London – a good, sound, easily understood book covering the basic methods in statistics. Smaller and cheaper than the ones above, so a useful first text.

Campbell, M. J. (2001) *Statistics at Square Two*, 2nd edn, BMJ Books, London – the companion book for *Statistics at Square One*, building on basic knowledge to include more complex statistical techniques.

Campbell, M. & Machin, D. (1999) *Medical Statistics, a Common Sense Approach*, 3rd edn, John Wiley & Sons, Chichester.

Bland, J. M. (2000) *An Introduction to Medical Statistics*, 3rd edn, Oxford University Press, Oxford.

Altman, D., Machin, D., Bryant, T. & Gardner, S. (2000) *Statistics with Confidence*, 2nd edn, BMJ Books, London.

8.3.2 Websites

There is a huge amount of statistical advice available on the internet. The sites listed below are a good starting point:

The Rice Virtual Lab in Statistics (http://onlinestatbook.com/rvls.html) provides *HyperStat*, an online statistics book, simulations and demonstrations, case studies and analysis capability.

John C. Pezzullo, a professor of pharmacology and biostatistics, has compiled a list of more than 600 links to web based statistical resources at http://statpages.org/. There are software packages to undertake analysis and also links to online statistics books, tutorials, downloadable software, and other related resources.

Bandolier has some good explanations of statistical terms: http://www.jr2.ox.ac.uk/bandolier/glossary.html

The Statistical Education through Problem Solving website is targeted at those who teach statistics but contains a comprehensive glossary: http://www.stats.gla.ac.uk/steps/glossary/index.html

Simple Interactive Statistical Analysis (SISA) includes a variety of resources including random number generators and power calculators: http://www.quantitativeskills.com/sisa/

Randomization.com provides random number generators at: http://www.randomization.com/

8.3.3 Papers

The *BMJ* publishes the series, *Statistics Notes*, which provide the latest views on appropriate statistical techniques to use in medical research. There are over 45 papers on various topics including the following, which all expand on topics covered in this chapter:

Altman, D. G. & Bland, J. M. (1994) Quartiles, quintiles, centiles, and other quantiles. *BMJ*, 309(6960), 996.

Altman, D. G. & Bland, J. M. (1995) Statistics notes: the normal distribution. *BMJ*, 310(6975), 298.

Altman, D. G. & Bland, J. M. (1996) Presentation of numerical data. *BMJ*, 312(7030), 572.

Altman, D. G. & Bland, J. M. (1996) Detecting skewness from summary information. *BMJ*, 313(7066), 1200.

Altman, D. G. & Bland, J. M. (1999) Statistics notes: variables and parameters. *BMJ*, 318(7199), 1667.

Altman, D. G. & Bland, J. M. (1999) Statistics notes. Treatment allocation in controlled trials: Why randomise? *BMJ*, 318(7192), 1209.

Altman, D. G. & Bland, J. M. (1999) How to randomise. *BMJ*, 319(7211), 703–704.

Altman, D. G. & Schulz, K. F. (2001) Statistics notes: Concealing treatment allocation in randomised trials *BMJ*, 323(7310), 446–447.

Altman, D. G. & Bland, J. M. (2005) Standard deviations and standard errors. *BMJ*, 331(7521), 903.

Bland, J. M. & Altman, D. G. (1994) Correlation, regression, and repeated data. *BMJ*, 308(6933), 896.

Day, S. J. & Altman, D. G. (2000) Statistics notes: Blinding in clinical trials and other studies. *BMJ*, 321(7259), 504.

Matthews, J. N. & Altman, D. G. (1996) Statistics notes. Interaction 2: Compare effect sizes not P values. *BMJ*, 313(7060), 808.

8.4 References

Altman, D. G. (1999) *Practical Statistics for Medical Research*, 1st edn. Chapman and Hall, London.

Hickson, M., D'Souza, A. L., Muthu, N., Rogers, T. R., Want, S., Rajkumar, C. & Bulpitt, C. J. (2007) Use of probiotic *Lactobacillus* preparation to prevent diarrhoea associated with antibiotics: Randomised double blind placebo controlled trial. *BMJ*, 335(7610), 80.

9 Successful grant applications

The next step, once you have sorted out your research protocol and have a clear plan of how to carry out the research is to get funding. A lot of small research projects can be carried out within work time, perhaps with help from students or volunteers, and no extra funding is required. Larger or more complex research is inevitably going to need finance in order to get it done.

If you do not require funding then you can skip this chapter and go straight on to getting ethical approval. Usually you would not apply for ethical approval until funding is guaranteed; ethics committees will expect to see what funding you have. Sometimes funders may ask for changes to your protocol; if you had got ethical approval first you would then have to go back to the ethics committee to get approval for your amendments.

Unfortunately, following all the advice here is not a recipe for automatic success – the competition for grants and other research awards is great. To be competitive your grant application must:

- Represent excellent quality research
- Be of value to health professionals
- Benefit patients
- Convince the judges that you can deliver the research
- Offer value for money (which is not necessarily the same as cheapness)

When writing your first application, read all the guidance you can find, take all the advice on offer and get someone with experience to read and critique your work. The most important thing to remember is that you will, at some stage, be rejected, so be prepared for it, and don't be disheartened. Rejections do not necessarily mean your project is not worth doing, but you do need to find the right funder and respond constructively to the criticism you have received.

9.1 Four keys to success

- Choose a funder that is likely to be interested in your work. If you submit patient oriented research to a body which funds basic science you are unlikely to be successful.

- Make contact with the organisation and get all the information you need.
- Write an application that communicates your intentions clearly. When you are writing, talk to your reader and remember they are not from your specialist field. You really have to sell yourself and your idea.
- Learn from your failures and keep trying. A big part of the research process is accepting criticism and learning from it. At all stages your work is constantly scrutinised and judged, and the grant application stage will be a particularly detailed examination. It is likely that you will be rejected and receive critical comments; try not to take these too much to heart and don't let it stop you trying again at another organisation.

9.2 Is it being funded already?

There is little point seeking funding if someone else is already doing similar work. You may have already checked the National Research Register (www. nrr.nhs.uk) to see who else is working in the same field as part of your literature review (see Chapter 4). It may also be worth looking at appropriate funders' websites to see what they have funded recently.

9.3 What funding is available?

Funding is available from a variety of sources including:

- Research Councils
- Government
- The EU
- Business and industry
- Charitable trusts and foundations

The best way to search for funding is to access the RDinfo database, available to all on www.RDinfo.org.uk. This lists all funding available to researchers in the UK. It can be searched by key word, type of funding or organisation. It also includes studentships, educational grants and travel bursaries.

9.4 Find out about the funder

Assess the potential funder by finding out as much as you can about their aims and objectives, their priorities, and their scope. Look carefully at what they have funded previously since this can give you a good idea of the sort of research they favour. Most organisations will present this information on their website. Some of the larger funders are listed in the resource section.

9.4.1 Make contact with the funder

If you can't find the information you need through the web don't be shy about ringing up and asking questions. Even if the organisation presents their information well on their website it is a good idea to try to make a preliminary contact at the organisation. Most grant giving bodies will assign someone to talk to potential applicants – they are keen to find good researchers to do their research. Once you make personal contact it will be easier to ring up to get extra information, advice or feedback after the judging process.

If you can't find the answers to the following questions in the literature provided it may be useful to make contact with someone:

▪ What do they fund? The web site will usually have this but it may be useful to discuss whether your project meets their criteria.

▪ What subjects or projects were funded last year? Again the website may have this, but discussing this will give you a clearer idea of what is likely to be funded.

▪ What are the future plans of the funder? Funders often have a theme they are following, which can change. If your idea doesn't meet their criteria now, find out whether it is something they might consider in the future.

▪ Who are the decision makers? It may help to know who is actually deciding on what is funded. This will usually be a committee with a variety of professions represented, but possibly not someone in your field. Knowing this will help you write the application in a style that will appeal to the decision makers.

On a more practical note you can also ask:

▪ What is the review process? This will generally be an external review by people working in the field you intend to investigate. It is useful to know how long the process takes and what the stages are.

▪ What is the deadline for submission? Give yourself sufficient time to meet it.

▪ How many people apply and what proportion get grants? This can give you an idea of the level of competition.

Most organisations now ask for a brief outline before you are invited to make a full application, and it is a good idea to do this even if it is not asked for. You want to make sure they are sufficiently interested in your idea before you spend weeks writing the application.

9.5 Patient involvement

The way research is done is changing. Traditionally researchers have pursued their own curiosity and tried to solve problems that they think are important. In today's research world it is increasingly important to involve members of the public. In Chapter 2 (Section 2.1.1) I highlighted the inclusion of patient involvement in the research governance frameworks for the UK. Funding bodies are also demanding more patient involvement. They want to pay for research that is relevant to people's needs and concerns and therefore more likely to be used. Thus, researchers have to change and learn how to involve the general public in developing their research. You will invariably have to explain how you have achieved public involvement in your grant application. Further details can be obtained from INVOLVE, an organisation with the specific purpose of increasing public involvement in research (www.invo. org.uk).

9.6 The application

Although most application forms will ask for similar information, they will unfortunately vary in format, order and detail. This means for each new grant you submit, you will have to reformat your work. Many large funders now have online application systems; other organisations will require you to fill in specific application forms to submit as hard copies. The first thing you must do is read all the guidance; I know I have said this before, but it is something people often leave until later and really waste time.

At this point your research protocol comes into its own (see Chapter 7 for details of protocol writing). You have already written the bulk of the application and it is now a process of cut and paste, and perhaps adapting the writing to an appropriate style. Write for an intelligent lay person, avoiding jargon and technical terms and always give a lay summary whether asked for or not.

Allow plenty of time for review and proof reading. It is vital to get other people to read your whole application to confirm it is clear, unambiguous, and can be understood by someone who is NOT in your profession. Writing an application is hard work and time consuming. At some stage you will almost certainly get bogged down in the details. Let your reviewers help you regain a clear view.

Remember you will also have to get a variety of signatures to confirm the support and approval of your manager, finance department, and other collaborators. You will need to allow several weeks before the closing date to do all this.

9.6.1 Important points to remember

Funders are looking to invest in good ideas and excellent researchers. They have the money, but they need the skills, expertise and experience to get the research done. Funders will give money when they find a proposal that fits their guidelines and shows good potential for success. Try to see it from the funder's point of view; why should they give you the grant?

Make sure your work fits the funder's guidelines. Take time to read through all guidance provided and make sure you are complying with all requirements. There is nothing more frustrating than spending hours completing an application only to find it will not be judged because something is missing. There can be a lot of information to read and take in, but time spent doing this is never wasted and will ultimately strengthen your application.

Write factually and definitively, focus on what you believe will happen. This is something many novice researchers find hard to do; they worry that what they hope to show will not happen and then they will be critically compared to their original application. Everyone in research knows that you are attempting to answer a question and that you do not know what is going to happen. Filling your application with words like 'hopefully' and 'possibly' makes you sound unsure and indecisive. Obviously there is a balance to strike; you should not make wild and unsubstantiated claims, but do try to write positively and with authority.

Although you are sending your application to an anonymous organisation, a real person will actually read it, so do talk to them in your application. The reviewers and judges are unlikely to be from your profession so make sure you avoid jargon and don't make too many assumptions about their background knowledge. Do not annoy the reviewers with poor grammar, spelling and long complicated sentences; it is hard work giving a fair review to a large number of applications so do make it easy for the reader!

Lastly, be really enthusiastic about your work; if you can't be then no one else will, and it will show. You have to sell it.

9.7 How you will be judged

Grant giving bodies get a huge number of applications and so the judging committees can be under a lot of pressure and time constraints. Imagine a committee with 40 applications to consider in a meeting which is scheduled to last 2 hours; this leaves only a few minutes discussion time for each application. You really have to make your application stand out and get the committee's attention.

The following are questions the committee may use to judge the application:

▪ What is the overall quality?
▪ How significant is the proposal in terms of its potential impact?

- ■ Are the aims realistic for the time and resources proposed?
- ■ How appropriate is the expertise of the applicants to the proposed research?

Make sure you have covered these areas clearly.

9.8 Acknowledgements

This chapter was written using information gained from attending a workshop run by Dr Philip Hills, Centre for Research into Human Communication and Learning, Cambridge.

9.9 Resources

9.9.1 Websites

RD Info is the key online directory to the research funding available to health and social care researchers. It currently holds information on over 1200 funding bodies and almost 4500 different awards. You can also register and request monthly reports of current grants in your area – http://www.rdinfo.org.uk/

European Community Research & Development Information Service (CORDIS) – http://cordis.europa.eu/en/home.html

INVOLVE is a national advisory group, funded by the Department of Health, which aims to promote and support active public involvement in NHS, public health and social care research – www.conres.co.uk

Major funder sites:

- ■ National Institute of Health Research (NIHR) – www.nihr.ac.uk
- ■ Economic and Social Research Council (ESRC) – www.esrcsocietytoday.ac.uk
- ■ Medical Research Council (MRC) – www.mrc.ac.uk
- ■ Biotechnology and Biological Sciences Research Council (BBSRC) – www.bbsrc.ac.uk
- ■ Wellcome Trust – www.wellcome.ac.uk
- ■ The Health Foundation – www.health.org.uk
- ■ Nuffield Foundation – www.nuffieldfoundation.org
- ■ Action Medical Research – www.action.org.uk
- ■ Stroke Association – www.stroke.org.uk
- ■ Research into Ageing – www.ageing.org
- ■ Dunhill Medical Trust – www.dunhillmedical.org.uk
- ■ Strategic Promotion of Ageing Research Capacity – www.sparc.ac.uk
- ■ Diabetes UK – www.diabetes.org.uk
- ■ British Heart Foundation – www.bhf.org.uk
- ■ Cancer Research UK – www.cancerresearchuk.org
- ■ Arthritis Research Campaign – www.arc.org.uk
- ■ The Leverhulme Trust – www.leverhulme.ac.uk

9.9.2 Books

Crombie, I. K. & du V Florey, C. (1998) *The Pocket Guide to Grant Applications*, BMJ Books, London – a helpful guide to the process and writing your application.

10 Obtaining approval for your research

Before you carry out any research you must get ethical approval to demonstrate that the project is not unduly burdensome to the participants and balances the risks and the benefits to the participants against the potential overall gain in knowledge. You must also obtain local Research and Development Office (R & D) approval to carry out the research at the proposed NHS site. University based research will not need the R & D approval but is likely to need approval within the university department. Both ethics and R & D processes are closely linked and will be considered together in this chapter.

A quick look at the history books demonstrates the need for a rigorous process to protect research participants (for example, look up The Tuskegee Syphilis Experiment, which only stopped in 1972). Atrocities that occurred during the Second World War resulted in the Nuremberg Code, which later led to the World Medical Association developing the Declaration of Helsinki in 1964. This remains the cornerstone of medical research ethics to this day (now in its fifth version, 2004, but currently under review in 2007). The declaration is a statement of ethical principles to provide guidance to those involved in medical research involving human subjects and can be read at www.wma.net/e/ethicsunit/helsinki.htm

The first question you might ask is: Since my research is so unlikely to harm the participants, why do I need to get ethical approval? The answer is that to date the research ethics process is the best way the medical community has found for ensuring that everyone follows the guidance given in the Declaration of Helsinki and carries out research with the safety and comfort of participants as the foremost priority. It is worth all the effort and the vast bureaucracy to avoid even one person suffering due to research activities. Nevertheless, there is currently pilot work on going to facilitate the fast track approval of those studies which obviously offer minimal risk to participants. Until this project is complete and deemed successful, all research, whatever it involves, must go through the current ethical approval process.

Obtaining ethical approval is relatively complicated and can take some time, but providing you break the process into a series of steps and carefully work through them you will be fine. All research ethics committees (otherwise known as RECs) have an administrator who will be able to provide guidance, and in my experience they are always very helpful; do not hesitate to contact your local REC if you have questions along the way. Only research projects require ethical approval and Chapter 2 explains what research is and how to distinguish between audit and service evaluation or development.

10.1 The two routes to ethical approval

There are two main routes for obtaining ethical approval: the National Research Ethics Service (NRES) and local university ethics committees. You must first establish whether you need to apply using the NRES or a local university system. If your project involves NHS property, staff or patients you need to use the NRES. Precise details of the remit of an NHS REC are given in Box 10.1; however, points (f) and (g) are open for review and may change. If you are a university based student or academic researcher, your project is based entirely outside the NHS and it involves only healthy human volunteers, you must use the local university system. In most cases the decision will be obvious but occasionally you may need further advice, in which case, ring your local REC officer who will be happy to help.

Box 10.1 Remit of the NHS Research Ethics Service in England. Department of Health (2001) *Governance Arrangements for NHS Research Ethics Committees.*

Ethical advice from the appropriate NHS research ethics committee (REC) is required for any research proposal involving:

(a) patients and users of the NHS. This includes all potential research participants recruited by virtue of the patient or user's past or present treatment by, or use of, the NHS. It includes NHS patients treated under contracts with private sector institutions

(b) individuals identified as potential research participants because of their status as relatives or carers of patients and users of the NHS, as defined above

(c) access to data, organs or other bodily material of past and present NHS patients

(d) fetal material and IVF involving NHS patients

(e) the recently dead in NHS premises

(f) use of, or potential access to, NHS premises or facilities

(g) NHS staff – recruited as research participants by virtue of their professional role

If requested to do so, an NHS REC may also provide an opinion on the ethics of similar research studies not involving the categories listed above, carried out for example, by private sector companies, the Medical Research Council (or other public sector organisations), charities or universities

---

The majority of this chapter focuses on the NHS ethics system but the principles will be the same for university systems. I aim to outline the main stages of the process to guide you through your initial contact with a REC. Figure 10.1 is a flow chart showing the process you will need to go through and each key decision point.

10.1.1 An introduction to the National Research Ethics Service

In 2004 the process for obtaining ethical approval within the NHS was standardised and governance was taken over by the Central Office for Research Ethics Committees (COREC), which is now known as the National Research Ethics Service (NRES). At the time of writing this book there are major changes being piloted for the NHS ethics approval process and there are two which will potentially benefit you as a researcher: the 'Early Provision of Advice' and the 'Fast Track of Studies Considered to Have no Material Ethical Issues'.

The pilot for 'Early Provision of Advice' was launched in May 2007 and is a screening process aiming to identify applications which are unlikely to meet the requirements of the REC, such as:

▪ Applications with poor presentation, which are incomplete, or have insufficient technical merit
▪ Studies submitted inappropriately (i.e. outside of the NHS REC's remit)
▪ Studies which may require further expert review in order for the REC to make a decision

The NRES then provides advice to bring the application up to an appropriate standard suitable for REC review.

The second pilot for 'Fast Track of Studies Considered to Have no Material Ethical Issues' commenced in April 2007. This pilot hopes to develop a filter system where all applications are examined by a small trained review team. This team will be able to give fast track approval to those applications deemed to have no material ethical issues and thus do not require review by the full committee. The results of these pilots are expected in early 2008 and may result in alterations to the ethics process.

The evolving nature of the NRES means that it is important that you refer to the website (www.nres.npsa.nhs.uk) in order to obtain the most up to date advice on the application process.

10.1.2 An introduction to university ethics systems

Unlike the NHS there is not a uniform system for ethical approval throughout the academic community. Each university will have its own particular process, but all will follow the same basic requirements as the NHS system

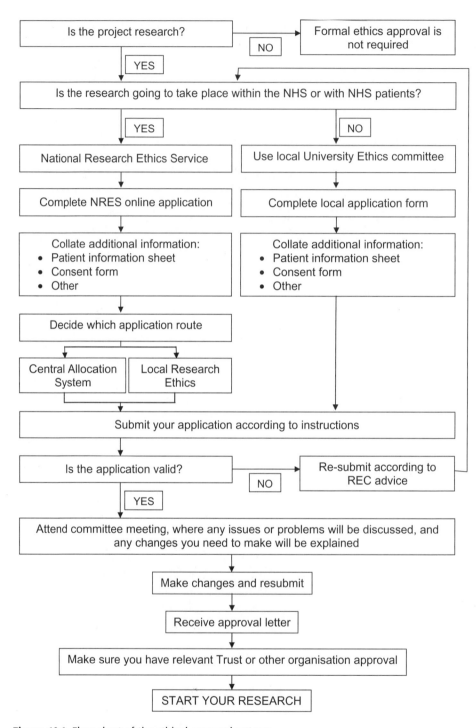

Figure 10.1 Flow chart of the ethical approval process.

described in the rest of this chapter. The specific procedure ↲ form will vary so you must obtain local advice.

10.2 The application form

The NRES use the same form for all studies and it must be filled in which requires registration at www.nresform.org.uk. Once registered can complete the form on any computer with access to the internet; you save work as you go along and come back to partially completed forms a later date. You can share the form with others to get their comments (a. long as they are also registered), and duplicate the form to create a person-alised template for future applications. The system also allows you to track your application and keep a record of all submissions made. The form is continually assessed and improved and the NRES are keen to encourage feedback from users to make the system as user friendly as possible. It has improved dramatically since the first version in 2004.

The first page of the NRES form is called the 'form sieve'; the answers you give on this page will dictate which further answers you will need to give. Once you have completed this page the main form will appear with irrelevant questions automatically filtered out. There are two sections to the form; Section 1 is the main form and Section 2 is for site specific informa-tion (SSI). The REC will review all sections but Section 2 will also be used for local R & D approval of the research project. If you have more than one site you will need to complete an SSI for each site in the proposed research.

University RECs will have their own application form but the type of questions asked will be similar to the NHS version. Whichever form you are using, work through systematically, completing all the questions you can on your first pass. Make a note of those questions that need more work or for which you need to ask advice and come back to them later. If you have a well prepared research protocol, most of this will be a process of cutting and pasting. There is plenty of advice on the NRES website about each question as well as detailed guidance on the whole procedure. The following general navigational tips will help you use the online form:

- At the top and bottom of every page there is a row of buttons for naviga-tion. The <navigate> button takes you to a list of all the questions so you can skip through the form.
- Your work is automatically saved every time you move to the <next> or <previous> page or click <save now>.
- When typing long answers click the <save now> button frequently. Sometimes it is possible to lose work because the internet connection 'times out'.
- It is usually better to type long answers into a word processor and then cut and paste into the online form.

■ Next to every question is an <i> symbol for question-specific advice – check this if you are not sure how to answer a question. If you get stuck or are unsure of what information is needed, contact the ethics committee administrator, your R & D office or a local Research and Development Support Unit if you have one (see www.national-rdsu.org.uk).

10.3 Confidentiality

Confidentiality is a big issue and you will need to include information about how your data will be kept confidential in your ethics application. You will also need to include statements about confidentiality in the patient information sheet. Advice on suitable wording is provided on the NRES website. The ethics requirements are designed to ensure you do not breach the Data Protection Act 1998, which is a set of rules to limit the use of personal information relating to living people.

Your research notes should be kept in a secure location such as a locked department or locked cupboard or filing cabinet. If you are unable to use a secure environment to store your notes with identifying patient details, such as consent form, letters with name, address or hospital number, should be kept separately to the clinical data collection forms, so that the data cannot be linked to the patient.

When creating your database for the analysis do not use the patient's name or other identifying information. Instead assign each patient a unique study number and use only this. Even though Hospital IT systems are designed to be secure and suitable to contain patient information, it is best practice to use only anonymous data.

It is customary to write to the patient's GP or consultant to say they are on a trial and to provide relevant information; indeed ethics committees expect you to do this. Make sure this is stated in the information sheet and the consent form, so the patient knows you are going to share their information in this way.

10.4 What else do I have to submit with the main form?

Along with the full application form you will almost certainly have to submit a patient information sheet and consent form. As a general rule written informed consent must be obtained from all research participants. Only in special circumstances are you likely to run research without written consent. To obtain informed consent you will need both a patient information sheet to explain your research and a consent form for the patient to sign. In addition you may need to submit other information to support and clarify your application.

10.4.1 Participants' information sheet

The participants' information sheet tells the participants what you are going to do, why you are doing it, and what you expect of them. Once you have completed the application form there is a temptation to sigh with relief and quickly put together the participant information. DON'T – this is a very important document that you must get right.

Give yourself plenty of time to do this carefully. Often all the queries and requests for changes from the REC relate to the information provided for participants. There are specific guidelines provided for writing this, since it must contain prescribed information. It will be sent back for changes if all compulsory information is not included. Comprehensive guidelines are given on the NRES website and even if you are using a university REC, these guidelines will be helpful to you.

Ask other researchers for examples of information sheets if you are not sure how to proceed. It can be particularly useful to use the wording from an information sheet that has already been approved, for example when describing the process for taking blood, using genetics information and so on.

10.4.2 Participants' consent form

The consent form provides the written evidence that you have gained the participants' explicit informed consent to include them in the research study. This makes it a very important document so I have devoted the whole of Chapter 11 to examining the issue of participant consent.

The NRES consent form also has a standard format and a template is provided on the website. An example is given in Figure 10.2. University RECs also frequently provide a standard template to use. Make sure all the points listed in the standard form are applicable to your research and consider if there is anything else that you need to specifically highlight to your participants, for example, if you intend to tape interviews and retain the tape for further analysis, or if you will retain blood samples for future analysis.

10.4.3 Other supporting information

You will also be required to submit other information to support your application. This will include, as a minimum, a copy of your research protocol and your CV. If you are a student, your supervisor will also need to submit their CV. Other documents that are commonly required include: copies of letters you intend to send to participants or intended participants;

(Form to be on headed paper)

Centre Number: 01
Study Number: (Ethics number given on submission)
Patient Identification Number for this trial: XXX

CONSENT FORM

Title of Project: **Study to investigate whether nutritional support increases muscle mass and quality.**

Name of Researcher: **Dr Mary Hickson**

Please initial each box

1. I confirm that I have read and understand the information sheet dated **DD/MM/YYYY** (version **n**) for the above study. I have had the opportunity to consider the information, ask questions and have had these answered satisfactorily. ☐

2. I understand that my participation is voluntary and that I am free to withdraw at any time without giving any reason, without my medical care or legal rights being affected. ☐

3. I understand that relevant sections of my medical notes and data collected during the study, may be looked at by individuals from [company name], from regulatory authorities or from the NHS Trust, where it is relevant to my taking part in this research. I give permission for these individuals to have access to my records. ☐

4. I agree to my GP being informed of my participation in the study ☐

5. I agree to take part in the above study. ☐

Name of Patient	Date	Signature

Name of Person taking consent	Date	Signature

When completed, 1 for patient; 1 for researcher site file; 1 (original) to be kept in medical notes

Figure 10.2 Example of a consent form using the National Research Ethics Service template.

copies of any recruitment posters or adverts you wish to use; copies of letters you will send to the patient's GP or consultant to inform them of this patient's participation; and any questionnaires or interview schedules that you intend to use.

The NRES system provides an applicant's checklist along with the main form that lists mandatory and other possible items you may need to submit (see the <checklist> button at the top of the page once you have opened your form). On first view this list may seem long and inexperienced researchers often feel compelled to include as much information as possible. Sponsors', statisticians' and funders' letters, referees' reports, and indemnity arrangements are not usually required in my experience for small local studies, provided you have given adequate information in the main form. A flowchart to describe the whole project can sometimes be useful if you have several visits or are studying more than two groups, but think carefully about whether such a diagram will clarify, or just serve to add another bit of paper to the ever increasing pile!

10.5 How to choose which REC to apply to

There are various routes into the NRES system, and the route you use depends on the type of research you are doing. For example, studies involving gene therapy, multi-centre studies, or studies testing a new drug will each require a different route. The NRES system can appear quite impenetrable and complex but you need to bear in mind that it is designed to accommodate the whole raft of research designs that are carried out in the UK, from large multi-centre drug trials to small observational studies. The key, as I said before, is to take it one step at a time and make sure you are taking the correct pathway before you move on to the next stage.

For the novice researcher the most likely scenario is that your research project will take place on one site only, will not involve testing medicines or medical devices, and will not be carried out on adults with mental incapacity or prisoners. If this is true for your project, you will need to apply directly to a REC in your local area. If this scenario does not describe your research you will need to use the central allocation system to be allocated a REC. You must check the NRES website for further details of this procedure.

To find a REC in your local area use the NRES website. From the home page enter the applicants' site and choose <contacts> from the left of the page. Use the <find your local REC> link and use the search tool to locate your most local committee. In theory, you can apply to any REC in the UK but I would suggest that you start with your nearest committee. If you find their meetings are fully booked try another committee near to you. The reason for this is that you are invited to attend the committee meeting to answer queries about your application, and clearly attending is most convenient at a committee that is quick and easy to get to.

10.6 The submission process

Once you have established the correct way to access the NRES and have contacted the appropriate REC you will be given a reference number which allows you an appointment in the committee meeting. From this moment you have four working days to actually submit your form, but if you have been following the preceding advice you will be ready now. You need to enter the REC reference number into the main form, check that it is complete and then lock it and the SSI form using the <manage/lock> links on the right hand side of the applications list. Once it is locked you cannot alter it and it is now accessible by the administrator of the REC. You must still print out one copy to sign and submit with your additional information as specified in the checklist. To print, open the form and use the <print> button at the top of the page – this does not actually print it directly, but allows you to download a pdf file of the whole document. Follow the on screen instructions to download it, and save it for your files.

10.7 What happens after submission?

After submission you will receive a letter from the REC confirming your application is valid and letting you know when the REC will meet to consider it. You are invited to attend the meeting and will usually have to phone up for a specific time. You do not have to go to the meeting, but I find it is helpful to be able to clarify points verbally with the committee and make sure that I properly understand what their concerns are; this makes responding afterwards much easier.

After the meeting you will receive a letter outlining the discussion that took place in the meeting (if you attended) and the items that require clarification. It is up to you to respond to this as soon as possible to ensure a prompt decision from the REC. On receipt of your explanations the REC will decide if they can now approve the project, although this decision is generally delegated to the chair of the committee to speed up the process. Providing you have answered all the queries satisfactorily you will then receive a letter giving you formal approval for the study.

10.8 Getting research and development approval

You are nearly there! Once you have ethical approval you need to contact your local R & D Office within your Trust for their approval. This process will vary between organisations so you will need to check locally. Once this approval is granted, you are free to start your project. University approved research may need further approval from your department, but generally, you can start once ethical approval is granted.

10.9 How long will it take?

Getting ethical and R & D approval can take several months, and if you need to make corrections or amendments to your protocol it can take much longer. You need to build this time into your research plan. Contact the ethics committees as soon as possible to find out the next few deadlines for submission.

There are rules that all RECs need to follow in assessing applications. The key ones as far as you are concerned are:

- All decisions must be given within 60 days from receipt of a valid application, but the time you spend answering corrections is not included in the 60 days.
- One ethical decision is valid for the whole of the UK.
- The committee may ask for clarification or further information only once.

As you can see, it is likely to take about two months providing there are no major changes to make and you are prompt in responding to the REC requests for information. However, I would say in practice to allow three months; there are invariably comments to respond to and an extra month in your research timetable will allow you to do this without adding extra pressure or letting your targets slip. If you are in full-time research (for example doing a student project) you have less excuse and should get your responses back immediately!

10.10 What happens next?

Once you have ethical and R & D approvals you are free to commence your research. Your approvals will be valid until the study is complete. However, you are obliged to submit reports on your progress and ask for approval of any amendments you need to make to your research protocol.

10.10.1 Changes once you have started

Once you have started your research project you may find you need to make changes. For example, to improve recruitment you may want to relax your inclusion and exclusion criteria. Any changes must be approved by the ethics committee *before* they are implemented. This is done using the substantial amendment form which can be found on the NRES website or by contacting your university committee.

An amendment is defined as something that happens after the trial has started, and, in my experience, substantial means anything other than very minor administrative details. The following examples would all require notification using a substantial amendment form:

▪ Someone new starts working on the project
▪ You change where you will recruit patients from
▪ You reword adverts for recruitment

10.10.2 Reporting to the ethics committee

You are required to notify the REC that approved your research of any serious adverse events that occur to patients on your study, which you think are related to any of the study procedures. This is done using a serious adverse event form. A serious adverse event is an untoward and unexpected occurrence that:

▪ results in death
▪ is life-threatening
▪ requires hospitalisation or prolongation of existing hospitalisation
▪ results in persistent or significant disability or incapacity
▪ consists of a congenital anomaly or birth defect

More stringent safety reporting is required for clinical trials of investigational medicinal products (in other words if you are testing a product that is classed as a medicine or a medical device), so if you are involved in this type of trial check the NRES site.

You are also required to submit annual reports to the REC until it is complete, and there is a standard form for the annual reports.

10.10.3 Finishing your study

On completion of the study you should submit an end of study declaration form and a final report. There is no standard format for final reports, but as a minimum, the REC should receive information on:

▪ Whether the project achieved its objectives
▪ The main findings
▪ Arrangements for publication and dissemination of the research
▪ Arrangements for feedback to participants

10.11 Resources

10.11.1 Websites

National Research Ethics Service – www.nres.npsa.nhs.uk.

Clinical Trials Tool Kit (Department of Health and the Medical Research Council) is designed to help guide researchers through the regulations of the UK Medicines for Human Use (Clinical Trials) Regulations 2004 and the EU Clinical Trials Directive in the UK: http://www.ct-toolkit.ac.uk/.

Medicines and Healthcare products Regulatory Agency (MHRA): Guidance on clinical trials with medications or health care products (includes some nutritional products) and how to get MHRA approval: http://www.mhra.gov.uk/.

The Patient Information Advisory Group (PIAG) was established to oversee arrangements created under Section 60 of the Health and Social Care Act 2001 – www.advisorybodies. doh.gov.uk/piag/.

Section 60 of the Health and Social Care Act 2001 – Guidance Notes can be found at www. dh.gov.uk/assetRoot/04/06/63/84/04066384.pdf.

Data protection Act 1998 – the Department of Health has useful guidance on this Act in the Policy and Guidance section > Organisation Policy > Records Management. A full copy of the Act is available at – www.hmso.gov.uk/acts/acts1998/19980029.htm.

Gene Therapy Advisory Committee (GTAC) is the UK national research ethics committee (REC) for gene therapy clinical research – www.advisorybodies.doh.gov.uk/genetics/gtac/.

The Human Tissue Authority – www.hta.gov.uk. This authority regulates the removal, storage, use and disposal of human bodies, organs and tissue from the living and deceased as specified in the Human Tissue Act 2004 (a full copy of this Act is available at www.opsi. gov.uk/acts/acts2004/20040030.htm). Scotland has a separate Human Tissue (Scotland) Act 2006.

11 Participant consent

As discussed in the previous chapter most research participants are required to give written informed consent. This is an extremely important part of the research process and you must understand the underlying principles of consent and the best way to approach the process.

11.1 What is informed consent?

One definition of informed consent is 'an ongoing agreement by a person to receive treatment, undergo procedures or participate in research, after risks, benefits and alternatives have been adequately explained to them' (Royal College of Nursing 2005).

There are three requirements that must be satisfied before a potential research participant can be said to have given informed consent:

- The consent should be given by someone with the mental ability to do so.
- Sufficient information should be given to and understood by the participant.
- The consent must be freely given.

It is also legally established that personal information should not be used for research without the explicit consent of the individual. This means they must have been asked specifically for their permission to disclose the information, been given an explanation of how the information will be used, and have given their permission in writing for the information to be used (Data Protection Act 1998).

Clearly it is important to ensure that those who take part in research understand exactly what is involved, and informed consent helps to ensure that people are not deceived or coerced into participating in research, and that the researcher has permission to collect and use the person's personal information.

11.2 Taking informed consent

You are not going to deliberately coerce or deceive people into taking part in your research project; nevertheless, subtle pressures may compromise the voluntary nature of consent. If a person does not have, or does not think they have, many viable options to choose from, this may place a pressure on them to participate. People may feel obliged to participate because:

- they do not know that participation is optional
- they think that participation is clinically recommended
- they think that if they don't participate, the care they receive will suffer
- they feel that they have a duty to help the researcher (possibly someone with whom they have an existing relationship) by participating
- they are not given enough time to consider their options (particularly if approached at a time of stress)
- they feel that unless they can provide a good reason, they may appear foolish if they refuse to participate
- once they have given their consent, and the study is underway, they do not realise that they are free to withdraw from the study at any time

Therefore, it is important to address these issues in the process of obtaining consent. A suggested procedure is outlined here:

- Talk through and explain the study in detail to the volunteer verbally, then provide the approved patient information sheet. You may also wish to go through the sheet with the patient or even read it out for visually impaired people.
- Take time to stress that participation is voluntary, their care will not be affected by their decision and that they do not have to provide a reason for not taking part.
- Be clear about the risks or inconveniences involved in taking part as well as the potential benefits for the volunteer.
- Make sure the volunteer has had time to consider the information fully and time to decide whether they want to take part; 24 hours is usually regarded as the minimum time. You must be satisfied that the volunteer has had sufficient time to consider his/her participation and ask any questions they may have.
- Look out for clues that a person may feel uncomfortable or are reluctant to take part; some people find it hard just to refuse. You must give them an easy way to say no, for example by suggesting they appear unsure and asking if they would rather not take part. An unwilling research participant is not going to help you complete a good study; it will simply result in more people dropping out or increased non-compliance.
- Before asking the volunteer to complete the consent form ask if they have any questions or concerns they want to discuss. Ask if they require any more time to think about it, or to consult their next of kin or another person. Again you must feel confident that the person fully understands the project, and particularly what will be asked of them during the study. It is in your best interest to take care over this stage, not only to protect the volunteer, but also to ensure your carefully recruited and assessed

participants don't drop out further down the line when their expectations are not met.

■ Ask the volunteers to complete the consent form themselves. The 'gold standard' is for each question or statement to be initialled; ask volunteers not to just tick the box. The form should be signed and dated by both the patient and the researcher.

■ The volunteer must be given a copy of the form. Either ask the volunteer to fill out two forms so they have a copy and you keep a copy, or photocopy the form for them.

Recruiting participants can often be difficult and as a researcher you are under pressure to recruit, but you must feel comfortable that all your participants have freely given their consent because you are responsible for the research and your participants' wellbeing. You need to achieve a balance between encouraging people to take part without coercion, and putting people off unnecessarily by focusing entirely on the risks and difficulties.

The problems of getting consent vary according to the type of study you are carrying out and the participants involved. Healthy volunteers may be influenced by financial reward to take part, whereas elderly participants may take longer to comprehend the details or be more vulnerable to coercion because they feel they have a duty to help. People with English as their second language or with low education or literacy may also need more time and simplified strategies to ensure understanding is complete (Sugarman, McCrory & Hubal 1998). Box 11.1 provides ideas to maximise your ability to get informed consent. You will have to think through these issues and highlight how you intend to ensure the consent process is robust in your ethics application.

A statement about how you intend to approach patients also needs to be included in the ethics application. Ideally potential volunteers should be approached in person, but this is not always possible. If you intend to write to patients or healthy volunteers to ask them to participate in your research,

---

Box 11.1 How to maximise your ability to ensure that consent really is informed.

Pick your time – when is the patient at their best?
Pick your place – find somewhere with no distractions, optimise the environment, and reduce clutter and noise.
Make sure the patient can see and hear to the best of their ability – use glasses and hearing aids.
Turn off your pager and mobile phone.
Simplify the consent process as much as possible.
Take time to explain the process, again and again if necessary.
Test that the patient has understood the key elements of the study (Sudore et al. 2006).

a copy of the proposed letter should be included in the ethics application form for approval.

11.3 Ongoing informed consent

Obtaining consent ought *not* to be viewed as a 'gateway event', after which a person's willingness and understanding may be taken for granted. Rather, it should be understood as an ongoing process that will continue for the duration of the subject's involvement.

A person's willingness to participate, and understanding of what it is that they are participating in, should be checked periodically, particularly if the researcher has reason to believe that one of these two essential elements of valid consent may have changed; for example, if the subject suggests that they are reluctant to continue in the project, or that they no longer understand some aspect of the research project pertinent to their decision to participate.

It is up to you as the researcher to ensure all your participants fully understand the project and if you have reason to doubt this you must discuss your concerns with the patient involved. I remember one patient who seemed to be getting increasingly disgruntled about what I was asking him to do, so I asked if he wanted to continue to take part but he repeatedly said he did. Nevertheless, he was clearly unhappy about participation and eventually I suggested it would be better for him if he ceased to take part. He seemed relieved and immediately cheered up; perhaps he just didn't want to let me down and so didn't feel able to make that decision himself. You need to be aware of these sorts of pressures and must always put the patients' needs first.

11.4 Taking consent from people who cannot give it

Taking consent when your volunteers may be cognitively impaired (for example they have learning difficulties or are elderly confused patients), unconscious, extremely ill or are children is difficult, and can pose some ethical problems.

The ethics committee will only approve the use of such volunteers in certain circumstances. You will have to justify why you need to carry out your research in this patient group and why it would be invalid to do the research in people who are able to consent. In October 2007 the Mental Capacity Act came into force, which gives specific rules for how to include incapacitated adults in research. The main ruling is that all research which includes people with mental incapacity must be approved by an NHS Research Ethics Committee; a university committee is not allowed to make such a decision. In Chapter 10 the process for ethical approval is described and all applications including such patients would go through the central allocation system. This is to ensure that the committee assigned to judge the application is trained to assess the research in view of the Mental Capacity Act.

The ethics committee can only approve the research if:

■ the research relates to the condition causing the mind or brain impairment, or to a condition resulting from or attributed to the mind or brain impairment
■ the research cannot be done as effectively using people who have full mental capacity
■ the research will produce results relevant to the condition (or a similar condition) affecting the person and have small risks or low adverse impact on the person, or it must have potential benefits to the person without disproportionate risk.

Of course in line with the view of informed consent as a continual process, the research must be stopped on the person if any of these criteria cease to be applicable.

The Act also indicates that before including the patient in the study, the researcher must consider the views of carers and other relevant people; respect any advanced decisions or expressed preferences of the patient; respect any objections the person makes during the research; and treat the person's interests as more important than those of science and society.

There is also clearer guidance in the new Act on how to obtain consent. Previously the named next of kin, other family members or carers were approached to give their assent for such patients to take part in research. (When agreement is asked from someone who cannot legally give consent, it is known as assent.) Now people who speak for the person who does not have capacity are referred to as a 'consultee'. A consultee can be a family member, carer or attorney, but cannot be a person paid to care for the patient or where they have a professional interest in the welfare of the patient. Importantly, a consultee with lasting power of attorney, makes decisions for the patient which have the same weight as if the patient made the decision. The consultee provides an opinion of what the patient would have wanted, so if they don't think the patient would have wanted to be part of the research they should not be recruited.

When it is clear the patient is confused, the procedure above is used. However, you may need to demonstrate that the patients you include do have the capacity to give informed consent. Thus, if you are recruiting from a group who could suffer cognitive impairment, for example elderly hospital patients, you need to test all participants for their mental capacity before deciding that the consent they have given is valid. Testing capacity includes consideration of three key questions:

■ Can the person understand the information you give them about the study?

- Can the person retain, use and assess this information?
- Can the person communicate their decision?

Assessing potential participants for their mental capacity is likely to include some sort of mental test, for example the abbreviated mental test score (Hodkinson 1972) or the mini mental state examination (Folstein, Folstein & McHugh 1975) plus discussion with the health care team. Usually consent is taken, then the test is carried out and if the volunteer does not pass the test they are immediately withdrawn from the study. Such test protocols would need to be described in the ethics application form for approval.

For people who are incapacitated but may regain capacity in the future, such as critical care patients, delayed consent can be used and this means informed consent is delayed until the patient is well enough to give it. The patient's relative or carer should still be consulted on the patient's likely wishes before data collection commences. However, data from such patients must be discarded completely should the patient not consent once they regain capacity. This procedure has been shown to fulfil the requirements of Data Protection Act 1998 and the Mental Capacity Act 2005 (Reid & Menon 2007).

11.5 Including children in research and obtaining consent

There is general agreement throughout the research community that research on children is needed. However, extra care is required in order to include children in research since childhood is a vulnerable time when any harm could have a serious impact. It is also important to make sure that children, as far as possible, understand and assent to any procedure they are asked to do. The Medicines for Human Use (Clinical Trials) Regulations 2004 state that written consent must be given by parents or those with legal responsibility for the child, but children should also be asked for their assent, if appropriate. For consent in other types of study, UK law remains untested, and the legal age of consent to take part in research (as opposed to treatment) is open to debate. If the child is able to understand the research proposal and what it would mean if they took part, they may consent for themselves. However, it is probably better to follow the Medicines for Human Use Regulations and always obtain consent from the parent or legal guardian as well as the child.

When recruiting children for research it is extremely important to provide information tailored for them in addition to the standard information sheet for the parent or guardian. Such sheets must take into account the child's age and stage of development. The National Research Ethics Service guidance suggests three possible age ranges which will require different information sheets: 11–15 years, 6–10 years, and 5 years and under. Thus, if you are recruiting children between the ages of 1 and 15 years you will need to design at least three information sheets specific to each age range. These will be much shorter and focus on the process of the research and how it will affect the child. They may contain pictures and must put the information in a context that the child can relate to. It may be that a printed information sheet is not suitable and a short video is a better way to convey the information to the child. It will be important to demonstrate to the ethics committee that you have developed such information with input from children of the appropriate age group.

11.6 Storing consent forms

There are clear guidelines for the correct way to store consent forms but your organisation may have additional local requirements. The original copy of the consent form, for any volunteer who is a patient at a hospital, should be stored in their medical notes. You can also retain a copy for your research files. Keep all consent forms and other forms containing identifiable data in a separate file from the data collection forms, and ensure they are secure.

If the person is a healthy volunteer or the research is taking place outside the health system the original remains in the researcher's files. In some hospitals healthy volunteers are given their medical notes to ensure there is a complete secure record of their involvement in the research, so you must check your local procedures. In all circumstances you must also give a copy of the consent form to the patient.

11.7 Resources

11.7.1 Websites

National Research Ethics Service (NRES) – www.nres.npsa.nhs.uk – look under Help 'Guidance' for information about research involving adults unable to consent for themselves and informed consent in general.

Data protection Act 1998 – the Department of Health (www.dh.gov.uk) has useful guidance on this Act in the Policy and Guidance section > Organisation Policy > Records Management. A full copy of the Act is available at www.hmso.gov.uk/acts/acts1998/19980029.htm.

Royal College of Nursing Research Society aims to promote excellence in care through research and development – www.rcn.org.uk/development/researchanddevelopment/rs.

11.8 References

Folstein, M. F., Folstein, S. E., & McHugh, P. R. (1975) 'Mini-mental state'. A practical method for grading the cognitive state of patients for the clinician, *J. Psychiatr. Res.*, 12(3), 189–198.

Hodkinson, H. M. (1972) Evaluation of a mental test score for assessment of mental impairment in the elderly. *Age. Ageing*, 1(4), 233–238.

Reid, C. L., & Menon, D. K. (2007) Time to get our acts together. *BMJ*, 335(7617), 415.

Royal College of Nursing (2005) *Informed Consent in Health and Social Care Research*. RCN, London.

Sudore, R. L., Landefeld, C. S., Williams, B. A., Barnes, D. E., Lindquist, K., & Schillinger, D. (2006) Use of a modified informed consent process among vulnerable patients: A descriptive study, *J. Gen. Intern. Med.*, 21(8), 867–873.

Sugarman, J., McCrory, D. C., & Hubal, R. C. (1998) Getting meaningful informed consent from older adults: A structured literature review of empirical research. *J. Am. Geriatr. Soc.*, 46(4), 517–524.

Part 2   Doing the research

You have designed your protocol, you have a grant to fund your research and your project has been approved . . . at last you are ready to start 'doing' the research. It is worth mentioning here that even though you planned your project in great detail it will not now just happen in a smooth and uncomplicated way. Research, and particularly human research, just isn't like that. Things will go wrong, the unexpected will happen, and you will get frustrated and stressed.

One of the most important things to remember is that if you are in doubt about anything – ask for help or advice. Do not battle on and hope things will sort themselves out, you will just end up in a worse situation; it is really important to address unforeseen issues as they arise.

The next three chapters cover collection of data, recruitment of volunteers and preparation and analysis of data. I have tried to highlight potential problems and offer practical advice to help you to avoid them.

12 Collecting your data

The data you collect in the course of your research will clearly be central to any conclusions you later make and so it is essential to take measures to make sure your data collection is accurate. Before you start recruiting participants you need to develop forms on which to collect the data, prepare the equipment you need to collect it, and design and prepare the database or software into which you will enter the data.

12.1 Confidential patient information

For each participant in the study you will need to keep a record of their name, address and other contact information. This can be recorded on a separate form, in a spreadsheet or simply entered into a note book. It is important to store this information separately from the participant's other data to protect confidentiality. I tend to keep one file with all the patients' contact information and consent sheets, and a second file for the data collection forms. A unique study number is given to each patient that cross references all the forms.

If you are dealing with large numbers of participants it makes sense to keep these records electronically on a spreadsheet. You will be able to keep patients' names, contact details and demographic details that affect inclusion into the study (like age, sex, or diagnosis) and record the outcome for each person you approach (entered study, ineligible, refused, unable to contact). If you are following up participants the spreadsheet will be a valuable tool to record when you contact them, why data couldn't be collected, and who has completed the study. Such a spreadsheet may look like Table 12.1. If you do this, make sure that you have noted it in your ethics application that you will keep such data and make sure that your spreadsheet is adequately protected to comply with the Data Protection Act 1998.

12.2 Screening form

For many studies it is useful to have a screening form, particularly if you have a large number of inclusion and exclusion criteria. The form is simply

Table 12.1 Example of a spreadsheet layout containing patient information.

Study number	Name	Address	Tel	Age	Sex	Entered study?	Reason for refusal or exclusion	Attended visit 1	Attended visit 2	Final follow-up call	Sent GP letter	Completed study (Y/N)
x	M. Smith	24 Howard Road, Smithton	Not available	64	F	Refused	Doesn't feel well enough	–	–	–	–	–
001	F. Jones	15 Beryl Gardens, Jonesford	12345678	45	M	Entered		Y	Y	12/10/07	Y	Y
002	T. Harris	Flat 3, 26 Harold Street, Harrisham	98765432	36	F	Entered		Y	N	20/10/07	Y	N

a list of these criteria so that each can be checked for the patient's eligibility. You will usually try to complete it before taking consent. However, some screening tests may themselves need consent and so you must delay screening until after consent has been obtained. For example, if you need to assess someone's muscle strength or blood cholesterol level as part of the screening process you will need to obtain consent first. On the other hand if your criteria relate only to age, where someone lives or whether they have used a particular service you can screen the patient before taking consent.

You are more likely to have numerous inclusion and exclusion criteria with quantitative experimental studies. Nevertheless, even if you have very few entry criteria it is still good practice to keep documented evidence that all entry criteria have been met. You may wish to include these on your data collection form, rather than having a separate screening form. An example of a screening form is given in Figure 12.1.

12.3 Data collection

Data collection in quantitative and qualitative research is very different and so requires quite different approaches. Qualitative data are collected using field notes as a supplement to any recorded or printed data. Quantitative data require a highly structured form. Both types of research need demographic data which are best collected on a structured pre-designed form.

12.3.1 Quantitative data collection forms

A good data collection form helps ensure the study is carried out according to the protocol. The following tips will help you collect the right data and carry out the study efficiently:

- Think about the order in which you will do your assessments and make sure the data collection form reflects this.
- Include all demographic and outcome data, as well as other influencing factors, as defined in your protocol.
- Include notes to aid your memory so you don't miss anything out, for example 'use the dominant arm for the hand grip test'; 'book the date for the next interview'.
- Give yourself reminders of tasks that need to be done, such as photocopying consent forms, writing to the GP, giving out instructions or equipment for tests.
- Include other aides-mémoire such as what colour blood vacutainer to use if you are taking blood, standardised protocols like rest the patient for 5 minutes before taking blood pressure, or phone or bleep number of the person to call if you have a particular problem.

Patient number.......................................

SCREENING FORM

Inclusion criteria:	YES

1. Out-patients 65 years and over with chronic respiratory disease. ☐

2. Recent reported unintentional weight loss of 5% or more in the last 3 months or a BMI <=20. ☐

Exclusions include:	NO

1. Patients with cognitive impairment as shown by AMT of less than 7. ☐

2. Taking nutritional supplements regularly in the last week. ☐

3. Taking fish oil supplements. ☐

4. Unable to attend follow-up appointments. ☐

5. Clinical signs of oedema. ☐

6. Concomitant confounding diseases (cancer, recent surgery, rheumatoid arthritis, unstable endocrine disease). ☐

7. Concomitant confounding drugs, including steroids prescribed within the last 3 months, or with a changing dose regimen. Patients who are taking low doses (e.g. 5–10mg) of steroids consistently for greater than 3 months can be included. Also stable doses of thyroxine. ☐

8. Greater than 1 month since last serious acute exacerbation of COPD. ☐

9. Has an allergy or intolerance to any of the supplement ingredients. ☐

Date patient signed the consent form...

Fish oil trial/forms/screening form doc   15/07/02

Figure 12.1 An example of a screening form.

- On every page include the patient's unique study number and date and use page numbers so you can tell if any sheets get lost.
- Try it out on the first 2–3 patients, and then make changes; design it to be easy to use.
- Ask yourself – could someone else pick it up, use it and get everything done correctly?

An example of part of a data collection form is given in Figure 12.2.

12.3.2 Field notes

Field notes are the way qualitative researchers tend to collect observational data and can be regarded as equivalent to the quantitative researchers' highly structured data collection form. Field notes are generally recorded in a notebook with much less structure but a systematic approach will produce more reliable and understandable data. The following tips from *A Data Collector's Field Guide* (Mack et al. 2005; reproduced with permission from Family Health International) will assist you in taking good field notes:

- Begin each notebook entry with the date, time, place, and type of data collection event.
- Leave space on the page for expanding your notes, or plan to expand them on a separate page.
- Take notes strategically. It is usually practical to make only brief notes during data collection. Direct quotes can be especially hard to write down accurately. Rather than try to document every detail or quote, write down key words and phrases that will trigger your memory when you expand notes.
- Use shorthand. Because you will expand and type your notes soon after you write them, it does not matter if you are the only person who can understand your shorthand system. Use abbreviations and acronyms to quickly note what is happening and being said.
- Cover a range of observations. In addition to documenting events and informal conversations, note people's body language, moods, or attitudes; the general environment; interactions among participants; ambiance; and other information that could be relevant.

12.4 Other forms and equipment

There are various other forms you may need depending on the type of study you are carrying out and the complexity of the study. If you are doing an interventional study, such as a randomised controlled trial, you will need somewhere to record adverse events and protocol deviations. If you

Patient number...

VISIT 1 – BASELINE (Week 1)

Date of assessment   _____

Demographics

Date of birth   _____

Sex   Male ☐   Female ☐

Ethnic origin   _____

Does the patient live alone?   Yes ☐   No ☐

Place of residence   Own home ☐

Other   _____

Medical history

Date of last acute episode   _____

Smoking habit   Never ☐

Ex - ☐   Date stopped   _____

Current ☐   Cigs/day   _____

Number of years   _____

Pack years   _____

Fish oil trial/forms/visit 1.doc   15/07/02

Figure 12.2 An example of part of a data collection form.

Patient number..

Anthropometric measurements

Weight (Kg) _____

Demi-span (cm) _____

Height (calculated from demi-span) (m) _____

BMI (kg/m^2) _____

If BMI =>20: % weight loss in last 3 months _____

MAC (cm) _____

TSF (mm) _____

Grip fatigue (seconds) _____

Hand used   Max grip strength (kgf) _____

Energy expenditure

RMR (kcal) _____

See Deltatrac report

Body composition

Does the patient wear a pacemaker? If yes DO NOT do this measurement

Yes ☐   No ☐

% lean tissue _____

% body fat _____

Water (l) _____

Impedance (ohms) _____

Bodystat Subject no _____

Fish oil trial/forms/visit 1.doc   15/07/02

Figure 12.2 Continued

are using a questionnaire to collect data this will need to be reproduced for use in your study or developed prior to starting the data collection. If you are using interviews or focus groups you will need to acquire recording equipment. It can also be helpful for all researchers to keep a diary or log of the research activities.

12.4.1 Adverse event forms

Adverse events are bad things that happen to the patient and can range from a minor ailment, like a muscular ache, to serious illness or death. The event may or may not be related to your research intervention but it is important to keep a record of any that occur, and the possible relationship to the intervention. You are required to report all serious adverse events to the ethics committee as described in Section 10.10.2.

12.4.2 Protocol deviations

When you run a study you will find that participants do not always do what you ask of them. This can be frustrating but is an inevitable part of human research. Often deviations from the required protocol will be very minor and may not matter much, but sometimes your instructions to participants are critical and failure to follow them will invalidate your results. For example:

■ If you need to take fasting blood samples and the volunteer has eaten breakfast, the test would be invalid and will need re-scheduling.
■ The subject may miss one or more appointments meaning some of the data are missing.
■ The subject may refuse to comply with some or all of the intervention.

In all cases it is useful to keep a record of what protocol deviations have occurred and why for each patient. This information can be extremely useful when you come to interpret the results. You may have a separate protocol deviation form or you can simply make notes on your data collection form when deviations occur.

12.4.3 Questionnaires and other data collection tools

Your study may require data collection through the use of a questionnaire. This could be a pre-defined one, validated to provide data on a particular issue. Examples include questionnaires to measure quality of life, nutritional status, physical activity, cognitive status, use of health resources, or economic information. There are numerous questionnaires available to use and it is generally better to chose one that has already been developed than create your own. When picking a questionnaire remember to consider validity and reliability. Alternatively, you may need to design and develop your own questionnaire. Of course you will have thought about this when planning your research so check the resource section in Chapter 7 for useful information.

Another common mode of data collection is to ask participants to keep diaries about usual daily activities where information on day to day variability is required. There are problems with this approach but it may help you to obtain information you cannot get any other way. Examples include diaries to record physical activity, emotion and mood, diet, or use of health care services. Problems centre on the honesty and consistency of reporting and serious biases are known to exist; for example overweight people tend to under-report what they eat, so use this strategy with care and make sure you understand the limitations.

Qualitative research often involves the recording of interviews or focus groups and requires the use of tape recorders and microphones. As with other equipment, your choice of what you use is likely to be limited to what is available in your organisation. Should you have a budget to buy new equipment do take advice from experienced researchers.

12.4.4 Research logs and diaries

Many quantitative researchers use logs to record their daily activities. This provides a written verification that certain activities have been carried out and can be used to confirm test or laboratory results. They are invaluable in verifying when and by whom particular findings were made. This may be a requirement of the organisation since such records can be essential if the research unit or project is audited. It may also be useful if the need arises to backtrack over events that have occurred to identify whether mistakes have happened. The important factor is that the log or diary is an unchangeable, dated record of research activity.

Qualitative researchers often use diaries in a more descriptive way to record in detail events happening during the research and also their own views, ideas, interpretations or feelings arising from participation in the research. The former are termed descriptive notes and the latter reflective notes, but both are regarded as part of the data collection and will inform the analysis. This does not have to be restricted to qualitative researchers; there is great value for all researchers in keeping a reflective diary. In particular, it is useful for people new to research since you will learn so much through the experience of carrying out a project. A diary will enable you to record your thoughts, experiences and new knowledge you acquire along the way. This will help enormously if you are undertaking research for a higher degree.

12.5 Design your database

There are various software packages that can be used to organise your data, but the most commonly used are Microsoft Excel or Microsoft Access. Excel is a spreadsheet application, whereas Access is a database application, which operates in a different way. Database software has distinct advantages for large complex datasets but is more complicated to learn. Spreadsheets, in particular Excel, are widely used, readily available and suitable for smaller datasets; so for the novice researcher this is likely to be the software of choice for data entry and management. Spreadsheets are extremely flexible but this lack of imposed structure can result in poor data entry and management. Here I focus on how to remain disciplined and structured in your approach.

When you set up your spreadsheet there are a number of key points to follow:

- If you are planning to transfer your data to a particular statistical software package to do the analysis, work out in advance how to do this.
- Rows are for subjects (patients or volunteers); one row per subject.
- Columns are for variables (weight, blood pressure, grip strength, sex, etc.); one column for each variable.
- Use the first row of the spreadsheet for the variable headings and make each heading unique, as short as possible, but readily understood.
- The first column should be the patient's study number – a unique number that identifies that patient only.
- All other variables should follow the order in the data collection form. This improves the accuracy of your data entry; when entering data you just follow through the form. You can always reorder the columns at a later stage if you need to.
- Each cell should contain only one value, and if you wish to use statistical analysis on the variable it is usually easier to use numbers not text.
- Code text by assigning a number (e.g. 1 = male, 0 = female) and use the numbers in your spreadsheet. Remember to keep a note of the coding you use.
- Explanatory notes can be included in your spreadsheet but add an extra column and use that for the text entry. For example, if the variable is weight but on several occasions you have missing data you may want to include the reasons in the database. You would use two columns – one for weight, which contains numbers only, and one for the reason for missing data, which contains entries only where weight is missing.
- If you have missing data always leave the cell blank. Do not add comments such as N/A or missing. Use the strategy above. Be careful about using '0' as the computer may include this as zero in any analysis. For example, if you use '0' for missing data in the weight column this will

be read as the patient weighed 0 kg. This is patently nonsense and will skew your analyses.

▪ Closed questions can simply be coded with a number for each possible answer.

▪ Open questions need to be categorised prior to analysis in quantitative methodology. Thus, you will group all the responses under a few headings and code each of them. For example, if you asked a question, 'What do you think is the best thing about undertaking a research project?' You may receive a range of replies but they could be grouped into the following headings:

☐ Gaining a more in-depth knowledge of a specific area = 1
☐ Increasing research related skills = 2
☐ Working with a different set of people = 3

Each of these headings is coded 1–3 and the code is entered into the database.

▪ Time related variables – one column for each time that the parameter is measured, so that blood pressure at baseline, mid-study and end of study = 3 separate variables.

▪ Use the power of computers. Don't do calculations the computer can do for you. Enter your raw data only and carry out all calculations once the data are entered. Thus, if you are interested in the difference between two measurements enter these two figures and then use the software to calculate the difference. This reduces error and saves you time.

▪ If you are using Excel use the data validation tool (check Excel help for details) to impose limits on the data you can enter where applicable. So if you have a category with only four groups you can set up Excel to only accept the numbers 1–4; entering any other number will result in an error warning message.

Figure 12.3 shows an example of a correctly laid out spreadsheet.

12.6 Code book

In order to make sense of your database and all these abbreviations keep a 'code book' – this could be a notebook (don't lose it!) or a Word document (better as you can keep a back-up). Alternatively, simply add this information into the spreadsheet; for example in Excel you can use 'comments'. Statistical software, such as SPSS (Chicago, IL), is structured to allow you to enter all this information directly into the spreadsheet and is one advantage to using such software.

Make sure you record the following:

▪ The abbreviated variable name and the actual full description of the data in that variable.

Microsoft Excel - example spreadsheet.xls

File Edit View Insert Format Tools Data Window Help   Type a question for help

C6   fx 53

Study No	F (1)/ M (2)	AGE (yrs)	Height (m)	date V1	Wt. V1	Waist_V1	HbA1c_V1	Gluc_V1	Chol_V1	date V2	Wt. V2	Waist_V2	HbA1c_V2	Gluc_V2	Ch
101	1	80	1.55	25.3.02	85.0	90.3		5.3	6.1	10.4.2	83.9	81.5	5.1	5.1	6.
102	1	50	1.74	28.3.02	119.7	103.0		5.7	4.2	22.4.02	116.2	108.8	5.4	5.5	4.
103	1	38	1.56	22.4.02	93.4	107.5		4.8	5.9	22.6.02	93.2	106.6		6.0	4.
104	1	44	1.62	26.4.02	97.3	99.5		4.7	4.8	22.6.02	96.1	99.6	5.0	4.6	4.
105	1	53	1.69	30.5.02	136.4	141.0	6.0	6.0	4.2	17.7.02	138.2	140.0	6.1	5.6	4.
106	2	61	1.93	12.6.02	142.0	130.0	5.2	4.5	4.0	17.7.02	142.5	118.8	5.1	4.5	3.
107	2	29	1.73	15.7.02	128.8	143.0	7.7	8.1	4.2	21.8.02	127.6	131.4	7.7	8.1	4.
108	2	32	1.85	22.5.02	122.4	128.0	5.6	5.9	5.4	24.6.02	123.5	122.5			
109	1	48	1.66	19.7.02	92.8	103.5	6.1	4.6	7.1	28.8.02	94.4	101.5		4.5	6.
110	2	29	1.7	8.5.02	110.4	106.5		4.5	6.0	5.6.02	106.2	110.0		4.6	6.
111	1	58	1.61	10.4.02	150.1	133.5		6.5	5.4	29.5.02	150.0	143.5	6.6	7.8	5.
112	2	68	1.75	22.8.02	162.3	150.4	5.4	5.3	4.6	2.10.02	162.3	148.0	5.2	4.8	4.
113	1	37	1.67	9.9.02	114.0	128.0	6.2	6.6	4.7	23.10.02	109.8	110.0	6.0	6.1	4.
114	2	83	1.73	14.10.02	109.4	130.5		4.5	3.4	20.11.02	106.4	101.0	5.6	5.1	3.
115	1	38	1.52	30.9.02	102.8	112.0	6.3	6.2	4.7	6.11.02	98.7	108.0		6.7	7.
116	1	61	1.6	7.10.02	90.7	88.0	5.5	7.0	3.3	20.11.02	91.4			5.8	2.
117	1	34	1.62	18.11.02	101.3	116.0	6.0	5.8	6.3	11.12.02	101.7	105.0	5.7	6.0	4.
118	1	70	1.63	28.10.02	99.2		5.7	4.8	4.1	15.1.03	99.4		5.6	4.4	
119	1	49	1.67	13.6.02	103.2	117.5	4.9	5.2	7.6	24.7.02	105.3			5.0	
120	1	73	1.65	27.6.02	150.0	134.5	5.5	3.9	5.3	11.9.02	149.5	134.0	5.1	4.1	5.
121	1	64	1.62	28.10.02	103.7	115.0	5.5	5.5	7.1	15.1.03	102.0	106.0	5.8	4.8	7.
122	1	55	1.67	16.10.02	107.0	119.3		4.9	6.6	4.12.02	108.1	118.0		5.0	7.
123	1	36	1.64	23.12.02	155.6		5.8		3.9	22.1.03	152.8				

MASTER IWM

Ready   NUM

Figure 12.3 The correct layout for a spreadsheet.

- The labels for all coded variables, e.g. male = 1, female = 0; no = 0, yes = 1, etc.
- Any additional information about the variable someone may need to understand, e.g. full question from questionnaire, or the units of measurement.

12.7 Preliminary data checking

I will discuss more about data checking and cleaning in Chapter 14 but it is worth stating here that errors can occur on the written data collection forms. These are hard to identify in later data cleaning and difficult to verify if you think there is an error. For example, the correct weight of a patient is 57 kg but when written it looks like 51 kg. Both values are entirely feasible and so will not be spotted in later data checks but could skew results. Thus, it is important to fill in data forms carefully and clearly. Spend a minute at the end of each data collection episode scanning the form for unclear data entry, missing data or any other errors. This is an important reason why clear, structured, well designed data collection forms are needed, and it is a job worth spending time on in order to save you time and effort later.

12.8 Resources

12.8.1 Websites

Statistical Services Centre, University of Reading, produce a series of guides:

- Data Management Guidelines for Experimental Projects
- Excel for Statistics: Tips and Warnings
- Disciplined Use of Spreadsheet Packages for Data Entry
- The Role of a Database Package in Managing Research Data
- Project Data Archiving – Lessons from a Case Study

See http://www.reading.ac.uk/ssc/publications/guides.html
   These are also included as chapters in a published book:

Stern, R. D., Coe, R., Allen, E. F., & Dale, I. C. (2004) *Good Statistical Practice for Natural Resources Research*. CABI, Wallingford.

The referenced book Mack et al. *Qualitative Research Methods: A Data Collector's Field Guide* is available free on the internet at: http://www.fhi.org/en/RH/Pubs/booksReports/QRM_datacoll.htm

12.9 Reference

Mack, N., Woodsong, C., Macqueen, K. M., Guest, G., & Namey, E. (2005) *Qualitative Research Methods: A Data Collector's Field Guide.* Family Health International, North Carolina, USA.

13 Recruiting volunteers

In this chapter I focus on how to recruit volunteers from both health care settings and the general public. I also discuss using publicity and writing letters to gain recruits for your research. Although cold calling is not used to recruit to health care research you may need to discuss the project over the phone, so I have included some guidance on this. Finally, I highlight the need to monitor and evaluate your recruitment by keeping good records. I discuss some of the problems I have encountered and the solutions I used, to provide you with ideas for how to go forward.

Recruiting volunteers for your research may be straightforward and it is often obvious how to go about it. But sometimes this is not the case and more thought is required on how to access different groups. Recruitment can make or break your study; a lack of people to include will make it impossible to complete the work. Novice researchers frequently overestimate the ease with which they can recruit and this is often the factor that inhibits the successful completion of a project. If you estimate that you can recruit 50 patients in 6 months but in reality you only get 25, you could be facing major difficulties. You may have to get more funding to carry on or be forced to finish the study with a reduced sample size and therefore end up with inconclusive results. For this reason it is extremely important to plan your recruitment strategy and monitor your progress closely; it is always better to address slow recruitment at an early stage.

In your research protocol you will have clarified who you want to include in your study using your inclusion and exclusion criteria. This may range from anyone who is healthy; healthy people but with specific backgrounds or experiences; any hospital patients; through to patients with specific conditions and who meet several other criteria. Generally, the more inclusion and exclusion criteria you have the more difficult recruitment will be. Equally, if you are exploring sensitive or difficult the topics, it will be harder to access suitable individuals and then to recruit.

13.1 In or out-patients from your hospital or health care unit

In some respects, recruiting from within the health care system is easier and less daunting than going out into the outside world and trying to find the right people. At least there are specific points of contact where people can be located, such as wards and out-patient clinics.

If you intend to recruit from wards or specific clinics you should first write to all the consultants whose patients may be involved to ask for their support and permission to approach their patients. This is a matter of courtesy and you should not expect any major objections if you have all the appropriate approvals.

13.1.1 Recruiting from out-patient clinics

In this context out-patient clinics include clinics in hospitals, GP practices, health centres or any site where health care clinics operate. You should always start by discussing the study with the person in charge of the clinic and the other staff who work there. They will need to know your inclusion and exclusion criteria so they can refer possible patients to you. These are very busy people and so you will need to make this decision process as easy as possible. For example, provide a simple summary of your criteria as a poster that can be pinned in front of the desk. If you have a long list of criteria only include the ones that concern their ability to refer you suitable patients, you can then check the other details. If you look at Figure 12.1 (p 120), the screening form lists numerous criteria, but my simplified version for the clinic only included patients with chronic respiratory disease, aged over 65 years and with recent weight loss or body mass index less than or equal to 20.

Clinic nurses can be great supporters of research work and they may also be asked to refer suitable patients, bleep or phone you so you can rush up and see patients, or generally just introduce the idea of the research to patients as they assess them.

If you work and treat patients in the clinic from which you intend to recruit, your job will be much easier. You will know the staff and the clinic process, and be able to access patients' notes to screen for suitable participants. If you do not routinely work in the clinic it is a good idea to be present whenever you are able. Patients can see you immediately, your presence will remind other staff to refer patients to you, and you can spend time chatting to suitable patients about the research. No one will explain and promote your research as well as you will. You will also be able to undertake any preliminary screening to make sure patients are eligible, provide patient information sheets and consent forms, and arrange follow-up phone calls to see if the patient does wish to participate.

You can also appeal to the clinic patients directly by using an advert or poster, giving brief details about the study, and a contact name and number to call if they are interested. Always try to include a benefit for the volunteers to take part in the study, for example, they get their cholesterol checked, they get the chance to discuss their experiences and opinions, or they may receive an intervention that may improve their health. If you are at a loss to find any particular benefit to the individual you can say they will be helping improve future patient care. Any posters or adverts aimed at research volunteers must be approved by the ethics committee, so if you didn't include a poster in your original application you must submit an amendment and get the wording and design approved.

If you know exactly what type of patient you are looking for (for example diabetic patients aged over 60 years) another strategy may be to search the clinic appointment lists on the hospital information system. You can then identify the people in the appropriate age range and send them the information on your study. Due to patient confidentiality you may not be able to do this yourself, but will have to ask the clinic administrator and consultant in charge to write to patients on your behalf. You will have to facilitate this by providing a suitable letter, appropriate inclusions such as a reply slip and pre-paid envelope, and paying for the postage if necessary. You will need ethics approval to write to patients so make sure you include this strategy in your ethics submission.

13.1.2 Recruiting in-patients

If your research involves hospital in-patients the first step is to decide which wards are most likely to be caring for the patients you are interested in. This could be obvious: if you are interested in an obstetric issue you will focus on these wards; similarly critical care patients will be on intensive care. However, recruitment could be more general, so for example, if you are examining referrals to rehabilitation wards, patients may come from any number of wards. Similarly, patients throughout the hospital could have the problem you are interested in, such as poor mobility, cognitive impairment, pain, malnutrition and so on. If your patient group is diverse and could come from many wards try to focus on a limited number, if you try to cover all wards it will be time consuming and unproductive. Ask the ward staff if they think their ward will provide suitable patients; they will know best what type of patients they care for. Then it is a matter of going round the wards and locating possible patients and approaching them.

Before you start, don't forget to inform the consultants and their teams that you will be recruiting patients under their care. Explain the study briefly, what is involved for their patients, and state that you have all the necessary approvals. They are responsible for each patient's care while they are in hospital so it is essential that they know what you are doing. Occasionally, some consultants will object to the inclusion of their patients and you will have to respect this; however, in my experience this is rare.

The study I ran looking at patients who were taking an antibiotic is a good example of how a recruiting strategy can develop. Clearly, patients taking antibiotics were spread throughout the hospital and in theory I could recruit from any ward. I started by thinking through the exclusion criteria and working out if certain wards would not be fruitful. Because immune compromised patients were excluded I avoided the intensive care wards. I also had to recruit patients within two days of starting an antibiotic so long stay wards were also of little use. I needed to exclude patients who had recent previous antibiotic treatment and after a short time I found vascular surgery patients often had a history of frequent antibiotic use so I avoided this ward too. After several months I had refined my recruiting strategy to a limited number of wards, including admission wards, care of the elderly and respiratory wards. I could then really focus on building relationships with the staff on these wards to make recruitment as efficient and rapid as possible. The key was to check all new admissions as soon as possible to find out if they were going on antibiotics. I tried numerous approaches including obtaining the previous day's admissions lists, liaising with emergency department doctors, asking medical teams on each ward to contact me if they prescribed antibiotics, and working with the ward pharmacists to highlight new patients. Many of these strategies failed, principally because people who work in hospitals are very busy and although they might want to help with research, it usually comes a long way down their priority list. The best way I found was to go to the wards and check personally with the staff there, and in the end this was the most time efficient and effective strategy.

In another study I worked on I was interested in recruiting patients just before they were discharged from hospital. Anyone who has worked in an acute hospital environment will know that predicting discharge dates is extremely difficult. Again the best way was to focus on particular wards, build up relationships with the ward staff and visit as often as possible. Finding time for a friendly chat or to help someone out paid huge dividends when it came to getting timely notification of someone going home.

13.2 Volunteers from the general public

Much health care research will involve people using the health care system, and hence volunteers can be recruited using the methods described in the previous section. Nevertheless, some research requires healthy volunteers or volunteers who are at risk of a particular condition but are currently not accessing the health care system. For this type of volunteer you will have to go out and recruit more widely from the community. There are several possible approaches that can be used individually or in combination, including advertising, writing letters, or publicising the research you are doing.

13.2.1 Advertising

Advertising in newspapers or with posters sited in work or public spaces can be an effective means of recruiting volunteers. You will need to investigate what is the best way locally and this may be a process of trial and error. If you know other researchers in the area, ask for advice.

Local papers may carry adverts; these will usually be at a cost, although some papers will provide free space for projects seeking volunteers (for example, the *London Evening Standard*). Ring your local papers and ask what they can offer you.

If you are using posters think about placing them in large offices, GP surgeries, sports centres, colleges, universities, or libraries. Before placing any adverts make sure you get the correct permissions to advertise and remember your advert or poster must have been approved by the ethics committee.

The group you are targeting will dictate the best places to advertise. For example, in the past I have looked for people who wanted to lose weight and a newspaper advert produced a large response. However, other studies requiring men with high cholesterol were harder to recruit for and we had to focus adverts on organisations with a high proportion of male employees, such as the police or fire service.

The following questions are worth asking when recruiting with adverts:

- How much will the advert cost? Have you got a budget for this? This comes back to effective planning; hopefully you will have included advertising costs in your research proposal and grant application. If you have no grant, your organisation may be able to help you, so discuss this with your manager or supervisor.

- Which is the most appropriate newspaper or publication to use? Think about the circulation and readership of the publication.

- What sort of response do you expect? The first time a colleague of mine recruited for overweight patients to take part in a weight loss trial she was inundated; the phone rang all day, which was unpopular with work colleagues! Make sure you have suitable facilities for dealing with the volume of enquiries you will receive.

- What extension number are you going to use? Who will have to answer the phone? Decide this in advance and if you are asking others to help with fielding calls make sure they know what information to get and what information to give out.

- Is there an answer-phone on this extension? If you are planning on using an answer-phone make sure the message is appropriate and gives clear instructions on what information to leave and when you will get back to the person.

▪ How are you going to screen people? Are there a series of questions you can ask to make sure volunteers are suitable? Adverts invariably attract a wide range of enquiries, from both suitable and unsuitable people. It will save you time to screen out the least suitable people on the telephone. Consider your inclusion and exclusion criteria and decide which ones you can ask the person about over the phone. Also consider what commitments the volunteer will have to agree to; spend some time explaining these to the potential participant and find out if they are willing to take on this level of commitment. For example, in the weight loss trial I ran, the volunteers had to attend six times over six months, have several blood samples taken, keep diet diaries and follow a specific diet. Despite large numbers of people showing initial interest in the trial many did not want to agree to this level of involvement.

13.2.2 Using publicity to recruit volunteers

Rather than advertising you can drum up interest in your study by telling people about it and then asking for volunteers. This could involve articles in magazines, newspapers or professional publications, interviews on radio or TV, or information on websites and leaflets. Each method has its own pros and cons, but whichever you use the approach largely depends on interested people being motivated to contact you. On one hand this means they are likely to be keen to take part in your research, but on the other hand you may miss a lot of people. Another bonus is that your research will reach a wider audience; it will raise your profile, and may lead to contacts with other researchers in similar fields.

Clearly, your study will need a strong public interest angle for the media to be interested in including articles about your project. For radio, TV and national newspapers or magazines your project is going to have to be large, novel and stimulate general interest. A good example is the Caudwell Xtreme Everest Research, which took place in 2007 and involved medics climbing Everest to look at blood oxygen levels; they used both radio and TV publicity to recruit volunteers. As a new researcher your project is unlikely to attract such large amounts of interest. Nevertheless, smaller local or specialised papers and magazines may well be interested. I wrote an article about one research project for the local paper aimed at older people, *The Pensioner*, which helped raise awareness of my research. It may have helped recruitment indirectly by making the work more familiar and recognisable; some people said they remembered reading about it and it made the idea of taking part more appealing.

Flyers and leaflets are an alternative to posters, with the advantage that people can take them away, or you can post them through doors. This is likely to result in fairly low recruitment rates but may access people you would not otherwise reach.

One major disadvantage of using publicity is that you have much less control over how your project is described and interpreted. It may well also attract unwanted contacts from people who aren't at all suitable for your research but still take up your time dealing with them.

13.2.3 *Writing letters*

To write letters of invitation to take part in research you first need access to the contact details of a pool of potential participants. With the legal issues now surrounding data protection this is not always easy, and organisations cannot always just hand over contact lists. Nevertheless, contact lists can be obtained via the electoral role or through databases developed to include people interested in taking part in research. An alternative is to ask organisations to send letters on your behalf.

If you are using letters the following tips will help:

- Make sure you spell the person's name correctly and use their correct title.
- Think about who the letter is aimed at and write in a style that suits this group.
- Compose a standard letter which introduces your research simply and clearly. Avoid jargon and write for the lay person.
- Use official headed paper as this will add the stamp of authority and approval to your study.
- Get ethical approval for your letter before you send it out.
- Use a suitable font size for the group you are writing to. If you are approaching an older age group consider those with visual impairment and use a large clear font.
- Look at the layout to make sure it is easy to read and doesn't put people off with a mass of text and little spacing.
- Make sure you include your name, address and contact details.
- Date the letter and tell the reader when you need a reply. Is it still worth them making contact, if they've not got around to responding until a month later?
- Check your spelling and grammar, and get someone else to proof read it.
- If you can, use a mail merge for producing your letters and the envelopes.
- Be clear about how the person should respond to you – is there a phone number to ring? Have you included a post paid envelope? Have you included a reply slip?
- Think about whether it is useful to include the patient information sheet with this introductory letter. You may find it is better to send this out only to the respondents who are interested and this could save a lot of paper.

Once you have sent out letters, as well as dealing with potential participants, you may also have to deal with queries, random questions, wrong addresses, and occasionally you may find you have written to someone who has died. This happened to me and I then had to cope with extremely distressed relatives who felt the hospital should have known about the death. Prepare yourself for these and any other likely scenarios. Make sure you know who to refer people to if they need more advice, want to access the health care system, or have some kind of complaint.

13.2.4 Phoning

You may not use cold calling as a method to make initial contact with potential research participants; it is regarded as too intrusive by ethics committees. You will need to send an introductory letter first (as described above) and explain that you will either:

▪ call unless you hear otherwise (know as an opt-out approach)

or

▪ ask them to respond so you can then call them (opt-in).

Ethics committees tend to favour the latter unless there are good arguments for why that might bias your sample.

When phoning people to try to recruit them or when talking to people who are interested the following tips will help:

▪ Prepare a script of what you plan to say to make sure you don't forget any important points.
▪ Introduce yourself clearly and make sure you are talking to the person you have called.
▪ Refer to your introductory letter and explain you are calling to discuss it in more detail.
▪ Confirm that the call is convenient to the person and if not arrange a better time to call back.
▪ If the person you are calling has not specifically opted in, check to make sure they are happy to talk to you. If not thank them for their time and finish the call.
▪ Explain your study in more detail, clearly describing what you want the person to do. You may need to say this several times and in different ways. Check the person has understood.
▪ Ask what questions they have, if any.
▪ Make whatever future arrangements are required.
▪ If the person is not there, be careful about leaving messages or discussing the study with another person. The usual approach to confidentiality should be taken. Do not discuss any details with another person. Leave your name, say it is about research, and that you will call back.

■ Be polite at all times. This may sound obvious and trite but when you feel under pressure to recruit people, or if you are short on time, it is easy to get tense and abrupt. You are trying to get people to help you so you need to be patient, listen to their questions and stories, remain positive and enthusiastic about the work and try to keep people focused on the issue you are discussing. Occasionally, you might come across people who are confrontational, angry or abusive; stay polite, explain you are going to hang up and put the phone down.

13.3 Keeping recruitment records

Data on your recruitment process are vital when you report your study, but it also enables you to critically assess the strategies you have used and plan a more effective strategy in the future.

For all recruitment you should keep a record of:

■ How many people were approached or responded to the advert
■ How many were excluded and why
■ How many were suitable but refused and why (if possible)
■ How many took part
■ How many later withdrew or were withdrawn by you and why

These data will show how difficult or easy it was to recruit for the study and can be included in the methodology when you write up the results. An example of how these data are used in writing up a study is shown in Figure 13.1. This information can be particularly valuable if your study is funded through a grant or commercial organisation and you need to account for your time and use of resources.

When you have problems with recruitment such as a higher than expected refusal rate or particularly slow recruitment, this information will help you decide how to change your strategy and improve recruitment. Information on why people refuse is always valuable and you should try to ask for this. Often it will simply be that the person doesn't want to take part, but there may be an underlying concern that you can address, either for that person or future people you approach. I ran a study once that involved providing older hospital in-patients with extra help with eating, drinking and nutrition in general. I didn't anticipate anyone would refuse since the intervention was so beneficial. However, many people did and when I explored the problem I found people were put off by the number of questions and assessments I was carrying out. To improve recruitment I offered all those who were not keen to agree to the full protocol the option of following a simpler protocol where we collected data on the main outcome measure only. This allowed me to improve recruitment and successfully complete the study.

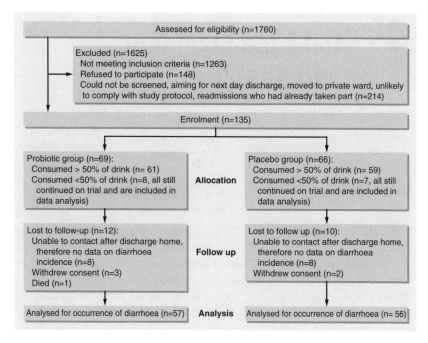

Figure 13.1 Flowchart of recruitment.

13.4 Informed consent

I have already examined the process of obtaining consent in Chapter 11 and I would recommend you go back and read this chapter before you start recruiting and approaching patients. Remember, as the researcher it is your responsibility to obtain informed consent; you must feel comfortable that every patient agreed willingly and fully understood all the implications of taking part.

13.5 Resources

Your best resources are your local experienced researchers. I have found very little information available otherwise.

Check with your professional organisation for local or national research networks, for example: National Physiotherapy Research Network (NPRN) and the local hubs – www.csp. org.uk/director/effectivepractice/research/nprn.cfm.

Also check with your local R & D office and Research and Development Support Unit (see Chapter 1 Resource section for details).

14 Data management and analysis

Once data collection is in progress the next stage of the research process can begin. This involves entering the data, checking and cleaning it, and carrying out the analysis. In this chapter I discuss data management and analysis in quantitative and qualitative research separately. Since whole text books can be written on this topic I have not set out to reproduce similar information here. I have aimed to provide a brief outline of the steps you need to take and provided some guidance for further sources of information in the resource section.

Undertaking analysis for the first time, in either type of research, will take you a long time; don't feel you are deficient in any way if the process takes significantly longer than you anticipated! It is important to take the time to get the analysis right, feel confident in your results and be able to defend them vigorously.

14.1 Quantitative research

Quantitative research follows a very structured, reproducible and definitive stepwise approach. With quantitative analysis your next steps will be:

- Data entry
- Clean and check the data for errors
- Carry out descriptive analyses
- Analyse the data to answer the specific hypotheses you have defined in your protocol (a priori analysis)
- Further analysis to explain results or to develop your theory (post hoc analysis)

14.1.1 Data entry

Data entry and management can be a full time job, and for large studies this task may be contracted out to companies specialising in this area.

However, for smaller studies you are likely to have to deal with your own data, using the software available in your institution.

Errors can be easily introduced during data entry and the following tips will help you to maintain accuracy:

- Enter data as you go along rather than waiting until you have collected it all; enter it as soon as you can after you have finished the data collection. Prompt data entry gives much more opportunity to re-check data if an error is spotted. Mistakes found a year after the patient finished the trial will be much harder to double check.
- It is dull and monotonous – so enter data little and often.
- A well designed database and data collection form will help keep the data entry accurate (see Chapter 12).
- Use features like validation and drop down lists in Excel to reduce entry errors.
- Make it as easy as possible to enter data; avoid having to type long names by using a numerical code as described in Chapter 12, Section 12.5.
- Enter data completely; do not leave forms half done and do not start until all the data on that form have been collected.
- Enter raw data and use the software to do calculations. This will be more reliable and accurate and is quicker than doing manual calculations during data collection.
- Software is available for double data entry; two people enter the data on separate spreadsheets, which are then compared for differences. Each difference can then be checked with the original paperwork. This reduces data entry errors and is particularly useful with larger datasets.

14.1.2 Clean and check the data

Before you start to analyse your data it is essential to check it for errors. Although this is a boring task it is well worth doing to prevent much stress and re-analysis later. The method includes looking for unfeasible data, extremes within ranges, and obvious errors in data entry.

For example:

- If you are recruiting people aged between 18 and 65 years you should not have any figures outside this range.
- If you have a categorical variable that you have coded (male = 1, female = 2) you should have no other numbers in this column.
- If you have measured a biological variable, check that the maximum and minimum are feasible. Heights over 2 m or under 1 m are highly unlikely to be accurate.
- Check dates for order – did your patient finish the trial before they started? This can be particularly important if you are looking at how long someone had a treatment or suffered a symptom.

■ For dates make sure you know what format is in use and if possible change it to one where there is no ambiguity, for example 10th December 2007 rather than 12/10/07.

To do these checks use scatter plots to spot outliers, filter tools to spot erroneous categorical codes and audit tools to check validation rules are met; and frequency tables can also be useful to highlight mistakes. The precise methods of using computer software to undertake these checks are not covered in this text; refer to the manuals of the software you are using.

Once you have found any errors you will need to return to your data collection form to check the correct value. If you continue to be suspicious that the value is not accurate, and it is possible, check with another data source, such as the medical notes or the volunteer. If the value remains ambiguous it becomes missing data.

14.1.3 Carry out descriptive analyses

This analysis describes the characteristics of your sample and examines the distribution of data. At this stage you may also identify potential errors highlighted by unexpected average or variation values.

For all analyses you need the number of responses and the number of missing data. If you have large amounts of missing data your analysis and results may be compromised. However, small quantities of missing data are almost inevitable and are usually not a problem (although it should be reported). Of course always try to avoid missing data if you possibly can during the data collection phase.

Next, you need to characterise and describe your study group. For categorical variables you need to look at frequencies. This will give you the numbers of cases in each category, such as how many males and females. For continuous variables you need to look at the central tendency and amount of variation (see Chapter 8, Section 8.1.4 for more details of these terms).

In order to carry out the next step of analysis, you will need to investigate how your data are distributed; do they have a normal (or parametric) distribution or not (non-parametric)? This tells you which tests are suitable for your data as previously discussed in Section 8.1.5.3.

14.1.4 Analyse the data to answer the specific hypotheses you have defined in your protocol

At last you are ready to actually test the hypothesis you originally set out to examine. When designing your protocol you should have considered exactly what questions you want your data to answer and what a priori analysis you will do. You must now choose the correct tests to do these analyses and answer these questions. Since this should all be pre-planned this should not pose too many problems. However, you will need to learn how to do the right analysis with the software you are using.

14.1.5 Further analysis to explain results or to develop your theory

Your data may throw up some other interesting theories or you may have got an unexpected result and want to do further analyses to investigate why. Be careful about excessive analysis. If you analyse any set of data enough, you will by chance alone get a statistically significant result sooner or later. Be clear about what you are trying to find out and do this analysis only.

Sometimes 'data dredging' can show interesting relationships but these are seen as 'hypothesis generating' only. In other words you now need to design a new study to test your new hypothesis.

14.2 Qualitative research

Data management and analysis in qualitative research also follows a structured series of activities. However, unlike quantitative research, the analysis overlaps with data collection and processing, and the data are repeatedly re-examined as the analysis progresses. As soon as the first pieces of data are collected, analysis can begin and the initial findings may alter the focus of future data collection. As the analysis progresses, further questions may emerge and new connections may be identified, together with a deepening understanding of the data. Earlier data is re-examined to explore it in the light of the most recent understanding of the data and to confirm new connections or theories. The steps involved vary depending on the author you read or the underlying philosophy behind your research design but the following are the main steps you will need to go through (based on Colaizzi's (1978) seven-step and Creswell's (2003) six-step process):

- Organise and prepare the data for analysis.
- Read through and gain a general idea of the content of the data and focus on the material that is important to the research question.
- Begin the detailed analysis by coding data into similar categories keeping focused on the data that pertain to the research question.
- The codes are examined in more detail and broader themes are developed in order to condense and reduce the data.
- An explanation or theory is then constructed around these themes and an interpretation of the data provided.
- Consideration is given to how the researcher's beliefs and experiences influence the analysis and to methods to validate the data.

14.2.1 Data entry and checking

For qualitative work data entry will initially involve transcribing recorded data, typing up field notes or scanning in documents or pictures. You can get professional help to do this, which will usually be more accurate and efficient. Nevertheless, there is a strong argument for you to transcribe or type up your own data, particularly when you are learning the research process; and in doing so you will become familiar with the data much more quickly.

Do preliminary checks on your raw data before transcribing to ensure the data are of sufficient quality to be useful. Transcribing is time consuming and costly so it is worth making sure your taped or written data are worth the effort. Once transcribed you may enter the text onto specialised software or choose to analyse it manually.

Qualitative data also need to be checked. Start by organising the data you have, so you know how much of each type of data you have, and you can identify the source of all the data, such as by individual, site or date. At this stage it is also useful to make sure you have back up copies of everything.

14.2.2 Doing the qualitative analysis

The first phase of qualitative analysis is to become familiar with the content of your transcripts (be it an interview, focus group or description of a discourse) and try to understand what the key messages are. As you read, the data will stimulate ideas and interpretations; make a note of these in the margins. Once you have a feel for the whole transcript, you can start to break the information down into specific quotes and begin the process of coding. At this stage it can be helpful to organise your findings in a tabulated form. Identification of common themes follows coding, and it is important at this stage to be clear how the raw data lead to the chosen theme. For example, the transcript may have several words and sentences about feeling frightened, anxious, concerned or worried; together these may suggest the theme of fear.

The above process is repeated for all the data, after which you can make connections between your themes, and link them together. Once you have achieved this essentially descriptive analysis, it is important to attempt to interpret the themes, using them to explain or understand the research question.

The process is one of construction, followed by deconstruction, followed by reconstruction. It is time consuming but also rewarding. Unlike statistical analysis there are no specific rules to follow; it is a creative process which is reliant on the thoroughness and skill of the researcher. It is helpful to read qualitative papers to provide an insight into what you are trying to achieve, and examples are given in the resource section.

14.3 Resources

14.3.1 Quantitative research

Also refer to Chapter 8 for further resources relating to statistical analysis.

14.3.1.1 Websites

Useful information about using MS Excel for statistical analysis – www.worldagroforestry-centre.org/RMG/ResMetRes/5/SSCExcel/index.htm

The Association of Statistics Specialists Using Microsoft Excel (ASSUME) – a wide range of articles, reviews, information and downloads about using Excel to do statistical analysis – http://www.jiscmail.ac.uk/cgi-bin/filearea.cgi?LMGT1=ASSUME&a=get&f=/welcome.html (or search for the association using Google)

Statistical Services Centre, Reading University – provides a series of guides on analysis to be found at www.reading.ac.uk/ssc/publications/guides.html. These are written for agriculturalists but the information is still useful and includes:

- Confidence and significance: key concepts of inferential statistics
- Statistical background to ANOVA
- Modern approaches to the analysis of experimental data
- Approaches to the analysis of survey data
- Modern methods of analysis
- Mixed models and multilevel data structures in agriculture

14.3.1.2 Books

Kinnear, P. & Gray, C. D. (2007) *SPSS 15 Made Simple*. Psychology Press Ltd, London.

Pallant, J. (2007) *SPSS Survival Manual*, 3rd edn. Open University Press Maidenhead.

Field, A. (2007) *Discovering Statistics Using SPSS*, 2nd edn. Sage Publications Ltd.

14.3.2 Qualitative research

14.3.2.1 Websites

Computer Assisted Qualitative Data Analysis (CAQDAS) Networking Project provides practical support, training and information in the use of a range of software programs designed to assist qualitative data analysis – http://caqdas.soc.surrey.ac.uk

14.3.2.2 Books

Miles, M. B. & Huberman, A. M. (1994) *Qualitative Data Analysis: An Expanded Sourcebook*, 2nd edn. Sage, London.

Boyatzis, R. E. (1998) *Transforming Qualitative Information: Thematic Analysis and Code Development*. Sage, London.

Lewins, A. & Silver, C. (2007) *Using Software in Qualitatve Research: A Step-by-Step Guide.* Sage, London.

14.3.2.3 Papers

Bailey, D. M. & Jackson, J. M. (2003) Qualitative data analysis: Challenges and dilemmas related to theory and method. *The American Journal of Occupational Therapy,* 57(1), 57–65.

14.4 References

Colaizzi, P. (1978) Psychological research as a phenomenologist views it. In *Existential Phenomenological Alternatives for Psychology* (R. Vallé & M. King, eds.). Oxford University Press, New York, pp. 48–71.

Cresswell, J. W. (2003) Qualitative procedures. In *Research Design: Qualitative, Quantitative and Mixed Method Approaches,* 2nd edn. Sage, London, pp. 179–207.

Part 3 Writing up and dissemination

The final stage is critical to the whole research process – if you don't complete this part you may as well not have bothered with all your hard work so far. Since research is about finding new knowledge and building on what others have found, it is vital to tell the world what you have added to the knowledge base. Others can then use this information to change how they treat patients, alter their service delivery or use it to plan future research.

This final section of the book covers what you need to consider when planning how to disseminate your research findings, and discusses the two most likely routes you will take to share your findings with others: presenting at a conference and publishing a paper in a scientific journal. The chapters also contain tips to help you write for journals and some of the etiquette involved in presenting and publishing your work.

15 Disseminating your results

I begin this chapter by discussing what you need to consider when planning the dissemination of your research findings, and underlining that successful dissemination is about more than simply presenting your work to your peers. Nevertheless, the two primary methods for initially disseminating your research are at a scientific conference and in a peer reviewed journal, so the second part of the chapter is devoted to describing how to achieve this. Whatever method you use to report your findings a clear writing style is vital. Therefore, I have finished this chapter with suggestions for improving the clarity of your writing.

15.1 Planning how to disseminate your results

Planning dissemination is really a matter of common sense and taking time to consider it properly. I have presented much of the information as questions for you to answer about your own work. This should provide the structure for you to develop a dissemination plan simply and quickly.

15.1.1 What information should I disseminate?

The first thing to consider is what you have found out. Be clear about this by asking yourself the following questions:

- What are the key messages from your results?
- Why are your results important? What do they add to what we already know?
- What action should be taken?

15.1.2 Who should I tell?

With this information you can start to consider how widely you need to disseminate your work and who is going to be most interested. Think care-

---

Box 15.1 Examples of groups and individuals you may wish to share your results with.

- Research participants
- Peers
- Other health care professionals
- Specialist team
- Patients
- Relatives
- Patient support groups
- Research funder
- Local managers

- Policy makers
- Directors
- R & D office
- Director of Research
- Your boss
- Students
- Local special interest groups
- International audiences
- Decision makers

---

fully about who will want to know about your results and don't just stop at the obvious (your manager, the R & D office and your peers). Think more widely to get your results really used (See Box 15.1 for further examples). Think about:

- What are you hoping to achieve by disseminating your research?
- Who will be interested in the results?
- Who can use this research?
- Who are the best individuals to target? Who can influence the group you are aiming at? This is particularly important if you want to change practice.
- Who can help 'spread the word' in a particular group?

15.1.3 How do I reach my chosen audience?

Once you have a clear list of the people and groups who need to know about your results, think about how to target the information to the audience. You may well have several groups you wish to inform, and for each group you will want to use a different emphasis. Consider carefully what the audience will want to know and how to tailor your messages to them. For example, you can inform your peer group through conference presentations or journal articles. To inform the patient group you may need to consider magazine articles, press releases or talks to patient support groups. Examples of different mediums to use to disseminate your information are given in Box 15.2.

Once you are clear about what information to tell to whom, you need to decide how to do it. Ask yourself:

- What activities will you undertake for each target audience?
- What tools or materials will you need to support these activities?
- When can you do it?

Box 15.2 Examples of methods of dissemination.

Conferences	■ Within your department or organisation ■ Area or regional meeting ■ Local, national or international ■ Posters ■ Oral presentation
Journal	■ Full paper ■ Short report or letter ■ News item ■ Editorial
Reports	■ To your funder ■ To your organisation's management ■ To key decision makers ■ Publish a report available to all
Teaching	■ Presentations ■ Workshops ■ Seminars
Lay press	■ Hospital newsletter ■ Local or national newspapers ■ TV and Radio ■ Magazines
Local meetings	■ Your own department ■ Your own multi-disciplinary team ■ Special interest groups within professions ■ Clinical governance or audit meetings
Professional press	■ Newsletters ■ Society magazines ■ Non-peer reviewed specialised press
Internet	■ Your own organisation's website ■ Relevant professional bodies' websites ■ Relevant patient groups or charity websites ■ Set up a specific website for the research

▦ Who in your research team is best placed to talk to this particular group?
▦ Have you got a budget for dissemination?

15.1.4 Evaluate what you have achieved

After carrying out your dissemination plan it is worth evaluating what you have achieved.

▦ Is it successful?
▦ Do you need to disseminate further or to different groups?

This seems obvious but often researchers are so relieved to get their paper accepted for publication or a poster presented at a conference, little work is done beyond that. Again the climate in the research world is changing and there is an increasing expectation from funding bodies to see detailed and effective dissemination of information, particularly information that will change practice.

15.2 Presenting at a scientific conference

One of the quickest methods of disseminating research findings to your peers and other health professionals is to present at a conference. The usual options available for presenting your original research are by oral or poster presentation. You may have the choice but frequently organisers decide after you submit an abstract (see Chapter 16, Section 16.1 for details of how to do this). Presenting at a conference is excellent for sharing preliminary results and also enables you to get early dissemination (publication takes many months). Try to submit your work to conferences that will publish the abstracts so you reach a wider audience than just the conference delegates. It is a great first step and should not be seen as second best to full publications. It is good for you because it can raise your profile and that of your organisation; it can also be fun and might even involve travel to exotic destinations!

If you are given the choice between a poster and oral presentation, be brave and opt for the oral presentation; this is seen as more prestigious and may give you a wider audience. Opting for the poster does not necessarily mean you will escape public speaking; you will frequently be asked to stand by your poster to discuss it, and many conferences run chaired poster rounds where you are required to do a very short (about three to four minutes) presentation of the poster. Chapter 16 covers preparing for a conference in more detail.

15.3 Publishing in a peer reviewed journal

The most important way to disseminate your work is to get it published in a peer reviewed journal. Writing a full paper requires more time, more substantial results and a large degree of determination and persistence. A thick skin and ability to take rejection are the essential characteristics of a researcher at this stage. Success is tremendously satisfying and your work is preserved for posterity, so it is well worth the effort. You will first have to make a judgement about whether your results warrant a full paper; if your study was a small pilot or your results are inconclusive a full paper may not be appropriate. You really need to obtain advice from a more experienced researcher, your supervisor or others in your research team.

Once you are sure a paper is the right step you will need to decide which journal you should submit to.

15.3.1 Which journal?

When choosing a journal you need to consider who you are aiming at and which journals cover the topic area. Ideally aim for a general journal with a wide readership, that is peer reviewed and has a high impact factor. However, your study may be in a very specific area and of limited applicability; this will mean you need to aim for a more specific journal. Similarly, if your results are confirmatory or simply adding slightly to the current knowledge, your work will be less likely to get accepted in general and high impact factor journals.

Be realistic, but aim for the highest impact journal you can. If you get rejected, you can then target a lower impact journal that is more relevant to your specific area. For instance, while the *BMJ* publishes only 7% of submitted articles, about 85% of rejected ones do get published elsewhere.

15.3.1.1 Impact factor

The journal impact factor is a measure of the frequency with which the average article in a journal has been cited in a particular year. The impact factor will help you evaluate a journal's relative importance, especially when you compare it to others in the same field. A higher impact factor means the journal is more widely read but likely to be harder to get published in.

To find out the impact factor of any journal use the Citation Reports produced on the ISI Web of Knowledge (http://portal.isiknowledge.com). Your library should be able to help you access this, or ask other researchers how you can get access locally. Many journals now display their impact factor on their website and this may help you. Table 15.1 is an example of the impact factors for specialist rehabilitation journals (these are monitored annually and thus will change). At the bottom of the table you will see entries from the 'general and internal medicine' category which are the highest impact factor journals within medicine. You will see from these examples how specialist journals tend to be rated much lower than general journals.

15.3.2 Types of submission

There are several types of submissions you may wish to use for your research. Each journal will differ slightly in what they accept so you must check the authors' guidelines for the details. The three commonest formats you will encounter are:

Table 15.1 The impact factors of rehabilitation journals in September 2007 (Journal Citation Reports, ISI Web of Knowledge).

Rank	Journal title	Impact factor
	REHABILITATION	
1	*Neurorehabilitation and Neural Repair*	2.403
2	*Journal of Rehabilitation Medicine*	2.168
3	*Manual Therapy*	1.931
4	*Supportive Care in Cancer*	1.905
5	*IEEE Transactions on Neural Systems and Rehabilitation Engineering*	1.842
	MEDICINE, GENERAL & INTERNAL	
1	*New England Journal of Medicine*	51.296
2	*Lancet*	25.800
3	*Journal of the American Medical Association*	23.175
7	*British Medical Journal*	9.245

- Full paper (around 2000–4000 words)
- Short report (around 1000–1500 words)
- Letter or case notification, such as a criticism, comparison or an urgent submission

Chapter 17 covers how to write a full paper in more detail. Much of that chapter would also be applicable to writing short reports or letters.

15.4 Authorship

If you publish your research you must make sure you include as authors all those people who contributed to the project in a substantial way. Authorship can be a tricky issue since publications are often required for career progression. Research is a process that occurs in distinct phases and people may be involved at quite different times and provide very different input. At the end it can be difficult to work out what contributions merit authorship.

To avoid these problems be very explicit about who is in your research team and what role they will play. This should be in your research protocol (see Chapter 7). All your research team would normally be authors for any publication. If you ask additional people during the course of the research for further advice or help, be clear at the outset whether or not this will lead to authorship.

The *BMJ* states that authorship should be based only on substantial contribution to ALL of the following:

- Conception and design *or* analysis and interpretation of data
- Drafting the article *or* revising it critically for important intellectual content
- Final approval of the version to be published.

This can offer a useful guide when deciding who merits authorship. Note that it is the intellectual contribution that is important. People who *only* collect data (however hard work that is!) are not usually authors, but certainly should be acknowledged.

The first author is often seen as the most prestigious position and is often assumed to be the person who has put in the most work; however, when working in teams this may be very difficult. Papers may be submitted with authors as joint first author but in reality someone has to go first in the list! There is no easy answer, but do sit down and discuss this at the start and decide as a team who that person should be. The first author usually writes the paper, co-ordinates comments and submits the final version – which can be very time consuming. If there are two or three people who have done similar amounts of work, it can help to think about who will benefit most from first authorship.

The final author in the list is also important and is generally the most senior person leading the team or the department in which the research is done. If you are new to research this is unlikely to be you, but do check within your research team who should have this position.

Finally, you should NEVER include people on your authorship list without first getting their permission and asking for their approval of the submitted paper or abstract. The content of the document reflects on all the authors and thus, they should all be given the opportunity to approve it.

15.5 Clear writing

Dissemination generally relies to a large extent on persuasive writing. Yet one of the most difficult skills to develop is that of writing clearly and concisely. Box 15.3 contains a list of things that colleagues have cited as making documents easy to read and Box 15.4 lists common errors to avoid. Whatever you are writing, think about your reader and make it easy for them to get your message.

15.5.1 Voice and tense

Use the active voice as far as possible, but always aim for the most concise way to get your point across. More information on active voice versus passive voice is given at http://owl.english.purdue.edu/handouts/grammar/g_actpass.html (or type 'online writing lab' into a search engine) but some examples are given in Table 15.2.

Box 15.3 What makes papers easy to read?

■ Clear organisation and use of sub-headings.

■ Logical order of the information.

■ Following a stepwise argument.

■ Using the active voice where possible (see Section 15.5.1 below).

■ Use the first person as appropriate – don't struggle to make everything impersonal.

■ Writing for the audience – but not assuming too much knowledge (people like a reminder!).

■ Concise writing. Don't say 'going through a development process' when you can just say 'developing'.

■ Consistent use of terminology and names. If something has several names or terms choose one and stick to it.

■ Consistent use of numbers. Always use figures for measurements with a unit (8 mmol, 6 years old, 10%). A good strategy for other numbers, unless instructed otherwise, is to write numbers under 10 as a word, and larger numbers as a figure. The only exception is in a list with other numbers (14 cakes, 12 buns, 9 biscuits).

■ Avoiding abbreviations and acronyms, but where they are useful always write the term out in full the first time. Abbreviations often help the writer more than the reader!

■ Choosing sensible abbreviations – a word is often better than a collection of initials, for example 'National Clinical Guideline on Management of Chronic Obstructive Pulmonary Disease' could be NCGMCOPD or 'the guideline'.

■ Clarifying the implications of the findings.

Box 15.4 What makes papers hard to read?

■ The writer assumes, 'because it is in my head, it must be in your head'
■ Jargon, technical terminology and buzzwords
■ Excessive abbreviations and acronyms
■ Long, multiclause sentences
■ Long paragraphs (this is visually daunting)
■ Long words where short ones will do such as 'implement' rather than 'do'
■ Waffle and wordiness
■ Incorrect spelling, punctuation and grammar

It is not possible to state a hard and fast rule regarding the tense you use. You would normally expect to use the present tense to describe results and conclusions that are still applicable. However, you would use the past tense to describe the methods.

Table 15.2 Examples of active and passive voice.

Active voice	Passive voice
The study examined the prevalence of . . .	The prevalence of . . . was examined in the study.
Most researchers acknowledge the difficulties of writing a great abstract.	The difficulties of writing a great abstract are acknowledged by most researchers.
Health professionals need to provide evidence for their treatments.	Evidence for treatments needs to be provided by health professionals.

15.6 Resources

15.6.1 Websites

Trent Research and Development Support Unit offers a useful resource pack on Presenting and Disseminating Research – www.trentrdsu.org.uk/resources_resource.html

Canadian Health Services Research Foundation – produces a useful set of Communication Notes (www.chsrf.ca/knowledge_transfer/resources_e.php) including:

■ Developing a Dissemination Plan
■ Reader Friendly Writing
■ Self-Editing – Putting Your Readers First
■ Dealing With the Media
■ Knowledge Transfer: Looking Beyond Health conference report, available in full at: www.chsrf.ca/knowledge_transfer/pdf/ktransfer_e.pdf

St. Cloud State University, Literacy Education Online provide advice on all aspects of writing – http://leo.stcloudstate.edu/index.html

Online Writing Lab gives advice on grammar and style – http://owl.english.purdue.edu/

Impact factor scores can be found on Journal Citation Reports, Institute of Scientific Information Web of Knowledge – http://portal.isiknowledge.com. Unfortunately, at this time this resource is not available to NHS Athens password holders. You will need to check locally how to access this information.

15.6.2 Books

Truss, L. (2003) *Eats Shoots & Leaves – The Zero Tolerance Approach to Punctuation*. Profile books, London.

Gowers, E., Greenbaum, S., & Whitcut, J. (1987) *The Complete Plain Words*, 3rd edn. Penguin Books, London.

15.6.3 Papers

Lavis, J. N., Robertson, D., Woodside, J. M., McLeod, C. B., & Abelson, J. (2003) How can research organizations more effectively transfer research knowledge to decision makers? *Milbank Q.*, 81(2), 221–222.

16 Preparing for a conference presentation

As I discussed in the previous chapter one of the two main ways to disseminate your research results are through conference presentations. It is a quick method of publicising your work and offers the chance to discuss it with other researchers in the field.

If your work is accepted for a conference presentation you, or one of your research team, will be expected to attend the conference to present it. Acceptance does not mean that the conference organisers will fund your attendance. Nonetheless, do not let lack of funding stop you submitting your work, as there are numerous small travel grants to support new researchers to attend conferences. Check the RDinfo website (www.rdinfo. org.uk) for available travel grants, ask the conference organisers if there is any support available or apply to your own or another organisation for support.

There are two options for conference presentations; a poster or an oral presentation. You may be asked for your preference or the organisers will decide which method is most appropriate. In order for the organisers to judge the quality of your work and its relevance to the themes of the conference you will have to submit an abstract summarising the work, which is judged prior to acceptance.

16.1 Submitting an abstract

You must first thoroughly read the guidance notes given by the conference organisers. This will tell you what format your abstract must be in, the word limit (usually about 300 words), layout preferences, submission deadlines and your responsibilities as a presenter.

An abstract is a succinct description of your work. It is NOT:

- A summary of the introduction – it is a summary of the whole piece of work.
- An extract of your paper – it must stand alone and be able to be read independently.
- Packed with references to other works – abstracts for conference submissions may contain a few key references only.

▪ An empty outline of what you intend to present at the conference – it must contain all the important information about your work.

A good abstract will contain:

▪ A good title – make it work for you. Set the scene and tell the reader what the abstract is about; it will tempt them to read on. Include key words but avoid abbreviations, jargon or ambiguous phrases.
▪ The purpose of the research – why did you do the study? What were you investigating? Why is this work important? What are you adding to current knowledge? Make sure you state your research question clearly. A good opening is often 'The purpose of this research is . . .'. Do not feel obliged to present all the findings from your study, especially if your study had several distinct objectives. Keep it simple and focus on one important area only.

▪ The methodology used – briefly explain the key points of your methods. This should not be a major focus of your abstract but you do need to include the design, setting, who you included and what intervention you used (if any). Say specifically what was done and how you did it, avoiding generalised comments.
▪ The results and conclusions – what did you find? What have you concluded? What, if any, recommendations can be made from these results? This is what most people are interested in so try to save most of your words for this section. It is acceptable in conference abstracts to include a table or a figure in this section and indeed this may be the best way to portray your results with the fewest words. Make sure you include the actual figures for your results not just the general trends.

A possible writing strategy is to write a concise and clear sentence for each of the bullet points listed above. Then count your words and see if you can add more. Use your extra words initially in the Results and Conclusions section, then in the Methodology. Next, edit and revise the abstract for clarity, making sure it flows together. Wait a day or two, come back to it with fresh eyes and edit again. Finally, ask a colleague who doesn't know much about the research to read it. They should be able to understand the key message without asking for extra information from you. Revise it according to their comments and suggestions, repeating the final step several times if you need to! The most important thing to keep in mind is to *make every word count*.

16.2 Preparing a poster for a conference

Posters are used at conferences to enable people to briefly present their work in a concise and time saving way. Posters are a visual presentation of the information, using pictures, graphs, and schematic diagrams as much as possible. Try to show visually what you have done and use text as little as possible.

Posters may be exhibited for the whole conference or just on certain days. People are free to go round the poster areas at any time but there are usually set times when you will be expected to be with your poster to answer questions or talk through the work you have done. Some conferences also expect you to do a very short oral presentation, standing by your poster during a chaired poster round. Check your instructions carefully for what you will be expected to do and prepare accordingly.

16.2.1 Planning your poster

The instructions will tell you what space is available to you, when you need to put the poster up and take it down, and any other specific requirements like minimum text size. You have already written your abstract, so you will have the foundation of your poster. You can add extra information on the poster as you are likely to have more space than the abstract allowed. Nevertheless, keep your poster focussed and only add extra information when it links very closely to the abstract text. For example, you may be able to include slightly more detail about the methods of your study.

Look again at your abstract and decide what your core message is. What is the main finding you want your audience to take away when they read your poster? Next, consider who your audience will be and design your poster with this group in mind. For example:

- Specialists only. You can assume a high level of knowledge about your area and safely use some jargon. Specialists in your field of study are likely to actively seek out your work and read it all. Your core message can be more detailed and specialised than for other groups. This situation is likely to be rare as most conferences cover a wide range of sub-specialisms.
- Wide-ranging disciplines within a broad topic. You can assume familiarity with the topic in general, but there are so many sub-specialities that jargon is best avoided and language kept simple. People in related fields will read your poster only if it grabs their attention, but since they will have a different perspective on your work they are worth making the effort to attract and talk to. In this scenario it is important to be clear and keep it uncomplicated, but make the conclusions and recommendations stand out as these might attract more attention. This is the most likely audience at most scientific conferences.
- Very general audience. You cannot assume any familiarity with the topic so you must explain everything in basic terms, avoiding technical lan-

guage. People in completely unrelated fields will probably not read the whole thing but may read the introduction and conclusion to glean the main points. Make it clear why you did the research and what the overall recommendations are. The reader's attention will be caught by the problem you are tackling and want to know how the results affect them. This is the type of audience you will find at conferences that are aimed at managers, decision makers and people who want to use research and put it into practice.

16.2.2 Creating your poster

You now have a good idea of the content and main message you are trying to get across. You also need to consider the space and layout; specifically do you need a landscape or portrait orientation? An important factor is what finance you have for printing and production. Your organisation may have a department who can assist with designing a poster and printing it professionally at no extra cost. You can have posters printed at high street shops or printers for a small cost if you do all the design work yourself. If you have no budget the simplest and cheapest way to create your poster is to write a series of A4 slides using Microsoft Powerpoint (or other presentation software) and then print and laminate them. The A4 sheets are really easy to carry around, (much easier than a poster tube) and changes can be made easily.

Establish early what your deadlines are and give yourself plenty of time to prepare. If this is the first time you have done a poster allow time to prepare it, edit it and fix mistakes. Your final deadline will be the travel date to the conference but remember your fellow authors will want to comment, you will need to make corrections and additions, printers need time, and the postal service may be involved too – so allow plenty of time to avoid stress.

16.2.2.1 What software to use

Presentation software is good to prepare a series of A4 slides as mentioned above. It can also be used to prepare bigger posters that you can then get printed elsewhere. Your organisation may have a standard template for you to use which will make the design process easier. Word processing packages can also be used to create a series of A4 sheets but are generally not useful for larger sizes unless you have a printer capable of printing the size you want. Spreadsheets (such as Microsoft Excel) will do simple graphs and bar or pie charts that can be pasted into the main poster.

Software comes and goes and gets improved so you may have access to other programs that are suitable to create large posters. Get advice and see what the best option is for you to use.

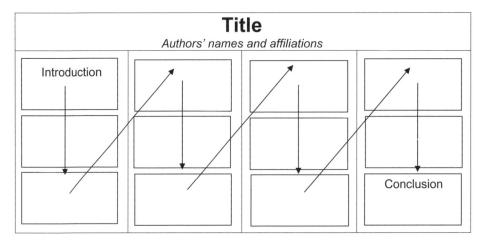

Figure 16.1 An example of the layout of a poster for a conference presentation.

16.2.2.2 Layout

Posters are best arranged as 2, 3 or 4 columns with the information flowing down, then across. A large title over the whole thing that can be read from about 10 m away is also needed. See Figure 16.1 for an example.

16.2.2.3 Text

Keep the text to a minimum and wherever possible use graphics instead. It is acceptable to use phrases and bullet points rather than full sentences. Use a simple clear font such as Arial or Times New Roman, and make sure you use 25–35 point for body text (including graphics) and 70–90 point for title panels.

16.2.2.4 Graphics

Pictures, graphs, figures and diagrams are all useful to communicate information simply and elegantly. Photographs are invaluable to show how something was done or describe the context of the research. Graphs and figures demonstrate relationships quickly but only if they are kept simple and clean, so stick to 2-D line graphs, bar charts, or pie charts, and avoid 3-D graphs unless you're displaying 3-D data. Flow diagrams are really useful to walk your reader through the process of the research or to describe a theory or mechanism.

All graphics will make your poster more appealing and eye catching but use with care since too many graphics can become confusing and destroy your simplified approach.

16.2.2.5 Colour

For reading ease use a light colour background and dark contrasting text. Avoid a dark background with light letters because this is more tiring to read. Stick to a theme of 2–3 colours only; any more will become fussy and overpowering.

16.2.2.6 Edit and evaluate

Once you have your first draft, re-read it and check it meets the requirements, then get someone else to check for errors. Edit ruthlessly to reduce text. If it's not relevant, remove it.

Don't forget to include your contact details so people who are interested can get in touch. Also give credit where it is due. Have an acknowledgements section, in smaller size type, where you acknowledge contributors and funding organisations.

Figure 16.2 shows an example of what can be done in presentation software to create a single slide that is then printed professionally as an A0 poster. Note that there is little text; it is mainly a table and diagrams, with a clear flow through to the conclusion. This could have been just as well done using a series of single A4 sheets.

16.2.3 Presenting your poster

If possible arrive early at the display site. Take a poster hanging kit with you – bear in mind, organisers try to have proper supplies but they often run out, and you then have to 'make do'. Nowadays Velcro fasteners are generally used, so take a supply with you or even better, stick them on the poster before you go.

Bring copies of a handout for your readers. It should include a miniature version of your poster and more detailed information about your work. You want people to remember you and your work, and of course be able to contact you. Put the handouts in an envelope hung with the poster and restock supplies periodically, if the poster is up for more than a day.

Make sure you're at your poster during your assigned presentation slot and have a 2–3 minute presentation prepared for people who ask you to talk them through the poster. This does not mean that you read the poster. Instead, give the big picture, explain why the problem is important, and use the graphics to illustrate and support your key points.

You may also be asked to present your work during a chaired poster presentation round. This means a group of interested people will go round each of a group of posters and listen to the author's explanation of the research. There is then time for a few questions and a discussion. This is a

Hammersmith Hospitals **NHS**

NHS Trust

Intensive lifestyle intervention combined with the choice of pharmacotherapy leads to weight loss and improvement in cardiac risk factors in the obese at 6 months, and maintenance of weight loss at one year.

J. Boyle and G. Frost, Department of Nutrition and Dietetics, Charing Cross Hospital, Hammersmith Hospitals NHS Trust, Fulham Palace Road, London W6 8RF.

Introduction

The rise in the prevalence of obesity over the last 20 years[1] has led to an increase in its related conditions such as type 2 diabetes and cardiovascular disease. Obese individuals who have successfully lost weight are prone to relapse at the end of a treatment programme[2].

Aim

• To investigate the effects of a 6 month lifestyle weight loss programme on weight and cardiovascular risk factors

• To assess whether this weight loss was maintained at one year.

Results

289 patients enrolled

33 active ongoing patients   175 discharged without completing

81 completed 6 month programme

46 followed up at 12 months

Anthropometry

	Start	6 months	% Change	P value
Weight (kg): advice + Xenical (n=23)	119.3 ± 25.7	108.6 ± 23.0	-8.9	<0.001
Weight (kg): advice only (n=58)	102.4 ± 18.3	95.0 ± 17.2	-7.0	<0.001
Weight (kg): combined group (n=81)	107.6 ± 21.9	99.1 ± 19.9	-7.7	<0.001
Waist (cm) (n=81)	111.6 ± 15.6	103.5 ± 14.1	-7.0	<0.008

Figures shown are the mean ± standard deviation

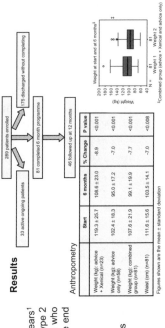

Weight at start and at 6 months[†]

†Combined group (advice + Xenical and advice only)

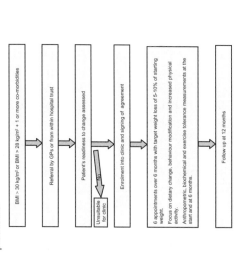
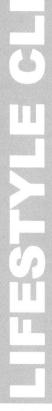

Figure 16.2 Example of a poster prepared using presentation software.
Thanks to Jo Boyle, Senior Dietitian, Obesity Management, Charing Cross Hospital. Presented at the Nutrition Society Summer Meeting in 2004.

fantastic learning opportunity where you can really get some objective feedback about your work, and discuss your findings with other researchers.

16.3 Preparing for an oral presentation

An oral presentation at a conference needs to be, like a poster, short and concise. You will probably have 5–10 minutes to present your work plus 2–5 minutes for questions and discussion, but you must check the conference instructions for the exact format.

Use specialist presentation software, such as Microsoft Powerpoint, to prepare your slides. Follow the guidelines I have given for preparing the content and design of your poster when preparing your slides. Probably the two most common errors people make with presentations is to have too many slides and hence go over time, or present slides with too much information on them.

As a general rule, allow one slide per minute – NO MORE – not even if you think you will skip over a few of your slides quickly. Prepare your slides with the minimum text and again give preference to graphics to get your message across. Plan and practise your talk carefully, including a dry run where you time yourself. This is particularly important if this is your first presentation at a conference, since a good experience the first time will give you confidence in the future. Good presentation skills can be developed throughout your career and you may already be competent and experienced in this area. However, if you are inexperienced I would urge you to attend training in presentation skills before your conference.

The most daunting prospect for novice researchers is the question and discussion section. People worry that they will be asked something they cannot answer and might look foolish. The first thing to remember is that you know more than most about your particular research area, therefore it is likely that you will answer with ease most questions put to you. Nevertheless, if you are new to research you may find researchers who will ask difficult and challenging questions. They are not trying to humiliate you (although occasionally some people do like to demonstrate their own expertise); they are genuinely interested in the work you have done. If you don't know the answer say so, add that it is an interesting question which you will have to investigate, but you would be fascinated to hear their view. Questions can be a tremendous learning opportunity, so try to view them this way rather than a test you might fail. Nowadays I would be disappointed not to get any questions and I associate a successful talk with lots of discussion.

The ideal way to prepare for any presentation is to practise until you feel comfortable and confident. Practise on your own first and develop some short notes to jog your memory as to what you want to say; do not write out your talk in full. Once you are happy with your talk get your research team and some colleagues together to hear you speak, give your presentation as if you were at the conference and then ask for questions. This will give you the opportunity to predict what people may ask and prepare your answers. Also ask for critical feedback: were all the slides clear? Did they follow the talk easily? Was it within the time limit? Could they hear and understand you? Were you speaking too fast?

You should be proud you have been chosen to speak at a conference because it reflects the quality and value of your work. Although you may be nervous, try to enjoy your moment of glory – you have earned it!

16.4 Resources

16.4.1 Websites

'Writing an Abstract', by Daniel Kies, Department of English, College of DuPage in the Hypertext book, Composition 2 – http://papyr.com/hypertextbooks/comp2/abstract.htm

'Writing the Abstract', in Millbrook House's open access site to support health professionals and students, University of Plymouth, School of Health Professionals – http://www2.plymouth.ac.uk/millbrook/rsources/litrev/lrabstract.htm

'Creating Effective Poster Presentations', by G. R. Hess, K. Tosney & L. Liegel – http://www.ncsu.edu/project/posters/

'Developing a poster presentation', by Jeff Radel, The University of Kansas Medical Center, School of Allied Health, Occupational Therapy Education – http://www.kumc.edu/SAH/OTEd/jradel/Poster_Presentations/PstrStart.html

Canadian Health Services Research Foundation – produces a useful set of Communication Notes (www.chsrf.ca/knowledge_transfer/resources_e.php) including

- Designing a Great Poster
- How to Give a Research Presentation to Decision Makers

16.4.2 Papers

Selvanathan, S. K., Udani, R. D., Udani, S. D., & Haylett, K. R. (2006) The art of the abstract. *Student BMJ*, 14, 45–88 (available online at http://student.bmj.com/issues/06/02/careers/70.php).

17 Writing a paper for a journal

One of the most satisfying parts of the research process is seeing your work published, and it really is worth the effort. This chapter aims to give advice on what to write in each section of your paper, in terms of structure, content and style. I also discuss how to approach the task of writing and include some additional advice on clear writing style. I finish by talking about what happens after submission, including reviewers' comments, acceptance and rejection, and correspondence about your work.

17.1 General advice

Every journal will have its own style and will give guidance on how to write and format a paper for them. Read and follow this carefully. Do not try to copy the final formatting you see in the published journal; this final version is the publisher's job. You should just submit a standard word processed document that meets the requirements they ask for.

The length of the paper will vary between journals, so check the guidance, but in general aim for around 3000 words (excluding references, acknowledgements and abstract). The longer it is, the harder it is to read and it will take up too much space, which will mean your chance of getting it published is reduced.

Chapter 5 discussed the critical appraisal of papers and it is worth revisiting this information before you start to write. Bear in mind what criteria others will use to judge your paper when it is published and make sure you have addressed all the potential areas for criticism.

Advice on choosing where you want to publish your work is given in Chapter 15, Section 15.3.

17.2 What goes in each section?

There is a fairly rigid format for writing a scientific paper, which includes title, abstract, introduction, methods, results, discussion, conclusion,

Table 17.1 A summary of the content of each section of a scientific paper.

Section of paper	Contents
Title	A succinct guide to the contents of the paper
Abstract	What did I do in a nutshell and what were the results?
Introduction	What is the problem?
Methods	How did I look at the problem?
Results	What did I find out?
Discussion and Conclusion	What does it mean?
Acknowledgements	Who helped?
Literature cited	Whose work did I refer to?

acknowledgements and literature cited. This format allows people to locate the information they need quickly and read the paper on a variety of different levels. Table 17.1 summarises the content of each section and the subsequent information provides more detailed advice.

17.2.1 Title page

Your paper should begin with a title that succinctly describes the contents of the paper. It should be short and unambiguous, yet be an adequate description of the work. Use descriptive words that you would associate strongly with the content of your paper: the patient group studied, the treatment, the location, the response measured or the key result. A majority of readers will find your paper via electronic database searches and those search engines frequently use key words found in the title. The clearer your title the more easily your paper will be found by others and then read – the whole point of writing in the first place.

You will also include the authors' names and institutional affiliations on the title page. Generally, the person leading the project and writing the paper will be the first author. If you are working in a team you will need to discuss this. Further advice on authorship was given in Chapter 15, Section 15.4.

You will also include in this section the name and full contact details of the corresponding author, who is the person the journal editor will communicate with, and will be the contact point for enquiries once the paper is published. You may also have to name the guarantor for the paper; this person accepts full responsibility for the work and the conduct of the study, has access to the data, and controlled the decision to publish.

Most journals will ask for your suggestions for key words (refer to Chapter 4, Section 4.1.1 for advice on choosing search terms; the same strategy can be used here) and a short running title, which can be published as a header at the top of every page.

17.2.2 Abstract

The abstract is one of the most important sections of your paper since it is what most people will use to decide whether to read the whole paper, and it will be freely available on websites and electronic databases. Since it is a self-contained summary of the whole paper always WRITE IT LAST.

An abstract with a full paper should have a similar content and be written in the same way as that described in Chapter 16, Section 16.1. However, there are a few issues specific to abstracts accompanying papers.

In a paper you will generally have a stricter word limit of only 200–300 words. This is partly because of the limits Medline and other databases place on the space allowed for the abstract, with anything longer being truncated. Since you will want the whole of your abstract displayed on these databases, stick to the limit.

In a paper an abstract should not contain:

■ references to other literature
■ abbreviations that are used in the full text – you must write it in full
■ any sort of illustration, figure, or table, or references to them

Once you have the completed abstract, check to make sure that the information in the abstract completely agrees with what is written in the paper.

17.2.3 The introduction

The introduction should establish the context of the work being reported. Do this by discussing the relevant research literature and summarising the current understanding of the problem you are investigating. Next state the purpose of your work in the form of the hypothesis, question, or problem you investigated. You can use statements like: 'The purpose of this study was to . . .' or 'We investigated three possible mechanisms to explain the . . .'. Briefly explain the rationale for the approach you have taken, saying why you have chosen to explore the problem in this particular way.

Do not include details of how you measured outcomes since this will be done in the methods section. However, if you are using a novel methodology the merits of this technique versus the usual method should be discussed briefly. For example, if you were looking at rheumatoid arthritis and hand function, and had developed a new way to assess function you might discuss the problems with current methods and why your new method is better.

The introduction should answer the questions:

- What was I studying?
- Why was it an important question?
- What did we know about it before I did this study?
- How will this study advance our knowledge?

The structure of the introduction can be thought of as an inverted triangle; the broadest part at the top representing the most general information and focusing down to your statement of purpose and rationale. A good way to get on track is to sketch out the introduction backwards; start with the specific purpose and then outline the scientific context, and then you'll have a good sense of what level and type of general information to begin the introduction with.

17.2.4 Methods

In this section you explain exactly how you carried out your study so another researcher could replicate the work. The following broad areas should all be included:

- Study design (such as randomised controlled, case control, survey, phenomenology, grounded theory).
- Subjects – the subjects used (age, sex, healthy or with a disease), inclusion and exclusion criteria, and when and where the study was carried out.
- Ethics – say what committee approved your study and whether you obtained informed consent.
- Demographics – say what information you collected about your subjects.
- Sample design – say how you selected your sample and the rationale for the sample size.
- Methods of data collection – say what you measured or what information you collected, how you measured or collected it and how often.
- Data analysis – for quantitative research say how the data are presented (for example, mean and standard deviation), how they were analysed and the statistical procedures used (a t-test was use to compare . . . , chi-squared tests were used to compare the categorical data . . .); include a statement of the level of probability at which you determined significance (usually at 0.05 probability). For qualitative research describe the analysis process and your rationale for using this method. You may also discuss researcher bias and validity problems.

This should be relatively simple to write because you have already written it for the research protocol. Be careful if you are only reporting one aspect of your study, and only include the information relevant to this aspect.

Organise the section so your reader will understand the logical flow of the investigation; subheadings can be useful, but check they are acceptable for the journal you are writing for. The purpose is to provide sufficient detail to allow replication of your work, but don't write the section like a manual. You can assume your reader has some knowledge of the area and the usual procedures used. When using a method described in another published source, you can save time and words by referring to it with the relevant citation. Always make sure you describe any modifications you have made to a standard or published method.

To improve the reporting of research, panels of experts have produced statements outlining the required content of reports of specific research designs. Examples include:

- CONSORT – randomised controlled trials
- TREND – non-randomised designs
- STROBE – observational epidemiology
- ORION – studies of nosocomial infections

Details of all these statements are given in the Resources section and if you are reporting any of these types of study it is worth complying with the statements' recommendations.

17.2.5 Results

The function of the quantitative results section is to objectively present your results *without* interpretation. This should be done in an orderly and logical sequence using both illustrative materials (tables and figures) and text. The text should guide the reader through the tables and figures by highlighting the answers to the questions you investigated, and providing clarifying information. Data which are presented in tables or figures should not be repeated in the text.

Prepare your tables and figures and then decide the logical order for them. Decide what each shows and include this in the text. Think carefully about the most appropriate illustrative material to use, such as bar charts, pie charts, tables or diagrams and decide which format suits the data. Do present the same data in different formats. Do not think whether you need a table or figure at all – you can present data in the text rather than creating a specific table, for example; 'The texture modified group had lower intakes of energy (3877 ± 400 KJ vs. 6115 ± 368 KJ, $p < 0.0001$) and protein (40 ± 6 g vs. 60 ± 8 g, $p < 0.003$) compared to consumption of the normal diet.'

Tables and figures should stand alone, in other words they must be understood without reference to the text. They need a heading, all abbreviations must be included in a footnote, and you should state the units and also what statistics are presented. For graphs or charts label the axis and include a legend.

Be careful about the use of the word 'significantly'. It has a specific meaning in relation to statistical significance. It is best to confine the use of this word to this context only to avoid confusion. However, if you include the p value in the sentence it is redundant to then include the word 'significant' in the body of the sentence. (The texture modified diet group had lower intakes of energy ($p < 0.0001$).)

Report negative results – they are important! If you did not get the results you anticipated, it may mean your hypothesis was incorrect and needs to be reformulated, or perhaps you have stumbled onto something unexpected that warrants further study. In either case, your results may be of importance to others, even though they did not support your hypothesis. Do not fall into the trap of thinking that results contrary to what you expected are necessarily 'bad data'. If you carried out the work well, they are simply your results and need interpretation. Many important discoveries can be traced to 'bad data'.

Qualitative research demands a slightly different approach since the findings are essentially the researcher's interpretation of the raw data. Include enough information to allow the reader to make a judgement about the claims you make from the data. Focus on the information that directly relates to your research question and try to avoid getting sidelined into other interesting theories. Make sure you back up every statement you make about your data with some evidence, such as quotations from interviews. If you have found contradictions or discrepancies in your data, do discuss these and don't skim over or exclude them. The logical sequence in qualitative research is to move from descriptions of any patterns you have found in the data to explanations of these patterns.

17.2.6 Discussion and conclusion

The function of the discussion is to interpret your results in light of what is already known about the subject, and to explain your new understanding of the problem after taking your results into consideration. The discussion will always connect to the introduction by way of the question you posed and the literature you cited, but it does not simply repeat or rearrange the introduction. Instead, it tells how your study has moved us forward from the place you left us at the end of the introduction.

Fundamental questions to answer here include:

- Do your results provide answers to your testable hypotheses or your research question? If so, how do you interpret your findings?
- Do your findings agree with what others have shown? If not, do they suggest an alternative explanation or perhaps an unforeseen design flaw in your experiment (or theirs?)
- Given your findings what is our new understanding of the problem you investigated and outlined in the introduction?

- Can you draw an overall conclusion from the work, perhaps how the results can be generalised or how your work increases the understanding of a particular process?
- Are there any recommendations for practice or policy?
- What would be the next step in your study or what future research is required?

Organise the discussion to address each section of the results and present this information in the same order as in the results section. Provide your interpretation of what the results mean in the context of the larger problem. Do not restate your results; simply remind the reader of the result being discussed by relating the result to the interpretation: 'The low energy intake relative to controls suggests that . . . (*interpretation here*). Be wary of mistaking the reiteration of a result for an interpretation, and make sure that no new results are presented here that rightly belong in the results section.

Subheadings can be useful to organise your presentation, and some journals will ask you to structure your discussion in a specific way. For example the *BMJ* encourages the use of the following structure which I find universally helpful whatever journal I write for:

- Statement of principal findings
- Strengths and weaknesses in relation to other studies
- Discussing important differences in results and meaning of the study
- Possible explanations and implications for clinicians and policymakers
- Unanswered questions and future research

It is useful to finish this section with your conclusions, which should summarise what you have discussed and be stated clearly and concisely.

17.2.7 Acknowledgements

If you received any significant help in thinking up, designing, carrying out the work, or in preparing the manuscript, or you received materials or funding from someone, you must acknowledge their assistance and the service or material provided. Provide names and what they assisted with; nothing more is required. Do check with the person you acknowledge to ensure they are happy to be named and there are no confidentiality issues.

Some journals have their own specific guidance on this topic, and may require you to list all contributors, including the authors, and to state what they have done.

It is also appropriate to acknowledge groups of people, for example ward staff or administrative staff who as a team may have provided general support. You may also wish to thank your volunteers.

17.2.8 Literature cited

This section lists the references that you cited in the body of your paper. Each journal has a different format and so it is important you check carefully that all your references follow the required format. The easiest and quickest way to do this is by using reference management software, which allows you to add your citations as you write, and then automatically creates a list at the end of the document in the style you specify. More information on referencing is provided in Chapter 7 Section 7.2.8 and on reference management software in Chapter 4, Section 4.2.

17.3 The writing strategy

First read Section 15.5 for tips on good writing style. The key to a writing strategy is to expect to write many drafts, since you will not get it right first time. After each draft self-edit ruthlessly and then once you have a half decent draft get others to edit and critically appraise your work.

One strategy to follow is:

- Write a draft you are reasonably happy with, but don't spend ages getting it perfect because someone else will change it! Make sure it roughly fits with the journal requirements.
- Circulate to the other authors and ask for comments.
- Incorporate the comments. You may need to meet and discuss it if there are areas of disagreement in the interpretation, or major changes to make.
- Re-write and circulate again for comments. This time, also ask someone outside the research team who is not familiar with the work, and is not in your profession.
- Once everyone is happy with the content and structure (you may need several re-drafts and this is normal!), go through to make sure it fits the journals requirements.
- Finally check the details. Are the references correct, are they cited correctly? Are all the authors' names and details correct? Have you included everyone you need to in the acknowledgements? Do all the tables and figures stand alone? Are all the numbers accurate? Is the abstract correct?

Allow yourself plenty of time to do this. A few days at least between writing drafts can help you come to it with a 'fresh eye', but in my experience writing a paper seems to extend over weeks rather than days!

Once you have your final draft ready and approved by all the authors you need to submit it according to instructions; this is increasingly through an online submission site. These are generally user friendly but not all allow you to save your submission part way through and come back to it.

Check the process before you begin and make sure you have all the information to hand. This will include suggestions for suitable reviewers, and information about ethical approval and conflicts of interest.

17.4 What happens after submission

Submitted papers are reviewed first by the journal editor who decides if the work fits in with the usual content of the journal. If this is the case your paper will then be sent out to be reviewed for its quality and content. At this stage you should receive a confirmation that your paper has been received and sent for review. If the editor feels the paper is out of the scope of the journal you will receive an immediate rejection.

Once the paper has been reviewed (this can take 2–3 months, and sometimes more) the editor will decide whether to accept your paper as it is, reconsider it after corrections or reject it outright. The latter two options are more likely. If you are given the chance to correct and improve your paper, read the reviewers comments carefully and try to comply with their suggestions. It is not always easy to take criticism of your carefully crafted masterpiece, and my advice is to read the comments and get cross; then forget it for a few days before reading them again in a calmer frame of mind! If reviewers haven't understood a paper it is usually because it wasn't written clearly.

When you resubmit always write a point by point response to every comment the reviewers made, linking your responses to the changes you have made in the paper. Do not feel obliged to make every change suggested; if you don't agree, argue your point of view and justify why changes are not appropriate. If you are unsure about certain comments do contact the journal editor for their advice.

If you are rejected you will be disappointed and this is often when new researchers give up. Give yourself time to recoup your energies then have another go. Rewrite the paper taking into account all the reviewers comments, then resubmit to a new journal. If you cannot address the comments you received you will need to think carefully about resubmission. You must get independent advice from a more experienced researcher. There may be a serious flaw in your work that has been missed and you need to decide whether the effort of rewriting and resubmission will be worth it.

It may take several resubmissions (my record is 3 different journals and 5 responses to reviewers' comments) but when you are accepted it is a great feeling of achievement. There are likely to be several more months before you see your paper in print and it will probably be published online first. Your work will be type set and you will have to proof read it before it can be published. Take time to proof read carefully as mistakes do occur.

Once it is published save a copy for your files, send round copies to all the other authors and don't forget to add the reference to your CV. If you are the corresponding author you may receive questions and compliments about the research, other researchers in the field may contact you and you may also be asked by editors to peer review papers on a similar topic. You are now published and have made a major step into the research world.

17.5 Resources

17.5.1 Papers

CONSORT statement – Campbell, M. K., Elbourne, D. R., & Altman, D. G. (2004) CONSORT statement: extension to cluster randomised trials. *BMJ*, 328(7441), 702–708.

Moher, D., Schulz, K. F., & Altman, D. G. (2001) The CONSORT statement: Revised recommendations for improving the quality of reports of parallel group randomized trials. *BMC. Med. Res. Methodol.*, 1, 2.

ORION statement – Stone, S. P., Cooper, B. S., Kibbler, C. C., Cookson, B. D., Roberts, J. A., Medley, G. F., Duckworth, G., Lai, R., Ebrahim, S., Brown, E. M., Wiffen, P. J., & Davey, P. G. (2007) The ORION statement: Guidelines for transparent reporting of outbreak reports and intervention studies of nosocomial infection. *J Antimicrob. Chemother.*, 59(5), 833–840.

STROBE statement – von Elm, E., Altman, D. G., Egger, M., Pocock, S. J., Gotzsche, P. C., & Vandenbroucke, J. P. (2007) Strengthening the Reporting of Observational Studies in Epidemiology (STROBE) statement: guidelines for reporting observational studies. *BMJ*, 335(7624), 806–808.

TREND statement – Des, J., Lyles, C., & Crepaz, N. (2004) Improving the reporting quality of nonrandomized evaluations of behavioral and public health interventions: The TREND statement. *Am. J Public Health*, 94(3), 361–366.

Gerrish, K. (2005) Getting published: Practicalities, pitfalls and plagiarism. *Journal of Community Nursing*, 19(8), 13–15.

17.5.2 Books

Hall, G. (2003) *How to Write a Paper*, 3rd edn. BMJ Books, London – a well structured book that is easy to dip into, taking you through from abstract to acknowledgments, with additional information on publishing.

Wager, E. (2005) *Getting Research Published – An A to Z of Publication Strategy*. Radcliffe Publishing Ltd, Abingdon, Oxon. – a useful reference text listing all you need to know about writing a paper from A to Z.

Albert, T. (2000) *Winning the Publications Game – How to Write a Scientific Paper Without Neglecting Your Patients*, 2nd edn. Radcliffe Medical Press, Abingdon, Oxon – another good reference book with an easy to read, accessible style.

Walcott, H. F. (2001) *Writing Up Qualitative Research*, 2nd edn. Sage, London – a text aimed at qualitative researchers, full of helpful advice and written with an accessible style.

17.5.3 Websites

Statistical Services Centre, Reading University – provides a series of guides to be found at www.reading.ac.uk/ssc/publications/guides.html including:

■ Informative Presentation of Tables, Graphs and Statistics
■ Writing up Research – A Statistical Perspective

STROBE statement – www.strobe-statement.org

CONSORT statement – www.consort-statement.org

TREND statement – www.trend-statement.org

Cabinet Office (www.strategy.gov.uk) allows free access to the following report:
Spencer, L., Ritchie, J., Lewis, J., & Dillon, J. (2003) *Quality in Qualitative Evaluation: A Framework for Assessing Research Evidence*. Government Chief Social Researcher's Office, London.

See Resources section Chapter 5 for other critical appraisal tools.

End note

I hope this book has inspired you to research a question and helped you carry out the project successfully. My motivation for writing the book has always been to enthuse people and to facilitate their progress from clinical practice into the world of research. I believe research underpins all professional practice and it is vital to identify, support and encourage those professionals who want to do research. I hope this book has made a contribution to this larger aim.

The results of your first project will undoubtedly lead to more questions and this may lead you to develop new, larger and more ambitious research projects. During the process of carrying out your first project you will have met other researchers, worked out what local procedures you have to follow and found people who are willing to help and support you. Now is the time to make use of these connections and create partnerships that will assist in furthering your research career.

The completion of your first project demonstrates you have the determination, enthusiasm and the right skills to be a researcher. I would urge you to use your energy and dynamism to further develop a challenging and stimulating career for yourself in clinical research.

Index